RHEOLOGY OF THE CIRCULATION

RHEOLOGY OF THE CIRCULATION

BY

R. L. WHITMORE
B.Sc., Ph.D., D.Sc., C.Eng., F.Inst.P.

*Professor of Mining and Metallurgical Engineering,
The University of Queensland, Brisbane,
Australia*

THE QUEEN'S AWARD
TO INDUSTRY 1966

PERGAMON PRESS

OXFORD · LONDON · EDINBURGH · NEW YORK
TORONTO · SYDNEY · PARIS · BRAUNSCHWEIG

Pergamon Press Ltd., Headington Hill Hall, Oxford
4 & 5 Fitzroy Square, London W.1
Pergamon Press (Scotland) Ltd., 2 & 3 Teviot Place, Edinburgh 1
Pergamon Press Inc., 44–01 21st Street, Long Island City, New York 11101
Pergamon of Canada Ltd., 207 Queen's Quay West, Toronto 1
Pergamon Press (Aust.) Pty. Ltd., Rushcutters Bay, Sydney, N.S.W.
Pergamon Press S.A.R.L., 24 rue des Écoles, Paris 5ᵉ
Vieweg & Sohn GmbH, Burgplatz 1, Braunschweig

First edition 1968

Library of Congress Catalog Card No. 68-18535

PRINTED IN GREAT BRITAIN BY A. WHEATON & CO., EXETER
08 003532 9

CONTENTS

v

PREFACE

SINCE the functional principles of the circulating system were established by the classic work of Harvey in the seventeenth century there has been steady progress towards a quantitative understanding of its dynamics and kinetics under normal and pathological conditions. Until comparatively recently it was usual to assume that the main elements of the circulation—the blood and the vessels in which it flows—behaved as simple liquids and solids respectively. But rheology, which is the science of the deformation and flow of matter, has taught us that most practical materials, including the constituents of the circulation, possess complex physical properties which affect their behaviour when a stress is applied to them so that they do not obey the theoretical laws applicable to simple solids and fluids. The object of this book is to show the extent to which rheological ideas are contributing towards a fuller understanding of the functioning of the circulation and to indicate areas in which advances may be expected in the future. It is intended to interest scientists trained in a range of disciplines who wish to appreciate developments in this field, and for teachers of biology or physiology seeking to interpret the biophysics of the circulation in modern terms.

The material is arranged so that the reader is first introduced to the basic rheological concepts and to the physical characteristics of the biological materials which compose the circulation. The behaviour of simple and complex fluids in motion is then considered and applied to the particular cases of plasma and blood. Experimental information on the dynamics of the circulation is then reviewed and discussed in the light of the known rheological properties of its constituents. Finally, the consequences of abnormalities in the circulation to its rheology are considered.

One problem in writing in an area which spans two disciplines is the terminology to be used. Not only may the two disciplines know the same phenomenon under different names but the same term may have different meanings to workers in the two fields. Care has been taken, therefore, to define the various terms when they first appear, the general practice being to use words in their scientific, rather than biological, sense whenever ambiguity is possible.

Interest in the circulation extends over at least 200 years and there is a formidably extensive bibliography associated with it. Rheological techniques, although of more recent origin, are also widely documented. In writing this book the policy has been to concentrate on the more recent work while ensuring that the references quoted are fully adequate to permit the reader to locate earlier work if desired.

Grateful acknowledgement is made to the Trustees of the Nuffield Foundation both for their sympathetic encouragement to work in an area which borders on science, engineering, biology and medicine, and for financing research aimed at filling some of the more obvious gaps in our knowledge of a new interdisciplinary field.

My sincere thanks are also due to my wife for her patient help in preparing the script and without whose assistance it would never have been completed.

SYMBOLS

A	Constant in eqn. (6.3).
a	Radius of a red cell.
a_1	Effective radius of a red cell.
b_1, b_2	Sub-axes of an ellipse.
c	Volume concentration of a suspension of particles.
$\bar{c}$	Mean volume concentration of a suspension of particles in a tube.
c_0	Maximum possible static volume concentration of particles.
c_c	Volume concentration of a suspension of particles flowing in a tube core.
c_f	Volume concentration of particles in a feed suspension.
$c_{\min}$	Minimum volume concentration of particles in a suspension at which a structure forms.
D	Rate of shear $= d\gamma/dt$.
$\bar{D}$	Mean rate of shear in a co-axial cylinder viscometer.
D_w	Rate of shear of fluid at a tube wall.
$\bar{D}_t$	Mean rate of shear of fluid across a tube.
d_c	Characteristic dimension in Reynolds number.
d_i	Internal diameter of a tube.
E	Young's modulus $= \tau_e/a$.
E_K	Elastic modulus of Kelvin solid.
E_M	Elastic modulus of Maxwell fluid.
f	Friction coefficient of a fluid in a tube.
H	Haematocrit (in per cent).
H_m	Minimum haematocrit for a yield stress to be present.
h	Height of inner cylinder of co-axial cylinder viscometer.
K_1	Constant in eqn. (1.11).
K_2	Constant in eqn. (1.12).
K_3	$\dfrac{R_2^2 - R_1^2}{R_1^2 + R_2^2}$ in eqn. (4.7).
K_4	Constant in eqn. (9.2).
K_C	Consistency constant in Casson equation [eqn. (1.8)].
K_{pl}	Consistency constant for power-law fluid [eqn. (1.4)].
l	Length of tube over which pressure difference is ΔP.
l_1	Calming length of tube after a junction.
ΔP	Pressure difference down a length l of tube containing a flowing fluid.
ΔP_w	Pressure difference across a wall.
Q	Flow rate down a tube of an unspecified fluid.
Q_B	Flow rate down a tube of an idealized Bingham plastic.
Q_C	Flow rate down a tube of a fluid obeying the Casson Equation [eqn. (1.8)].
Q_N	Flow rate down a tube of a Newtonian fluid.
Q_{pl}	Flow rate down a tube of a power-law fluid.
q	Quantity of fluid flowing in a tube annulus.
R_1	Radius of inner cylinder of a co-axial cylinder viscometer.
R_2	Radius of outer cylinder of a co-axial cylinder viscometer.
R_3	Radius of cone and plate of a cone-plate viscometer.
R_b	Mean radius of bend in a tube.
R_c	Critical radius for a Bingham plastic in a co-axial cylinder viscometer.

R_i Inner radius of a tube.

R_o Outer radius of a tube.

ΔR_o Increment in outer radius of a tube.

Re Reynolds number $= \dfrac{\bar{v}\,d_c\,\rho}{\eta}$.

Re_p Particle Reynolds number $= \dfrac{Re_t}{2}\left(\dfrac{r}{R_i}\right)^3$.

Re_t Tube Reynolds number $= \dfrac{\bar{v}_t d_i \rho}{\eta}$.

r Radius of a sphere.

r_f Radius of a concentric cylinder of fluid in a tube.

s Exponent constant for power-law fluid [eqn. (1.4)].

T Torque transmitted in a co-axial cylinder viscometer.

T_n Tension in an elastic solid.

t Time.

V Internal volume of unit length of a tube.

ΔV Increment in volume of unit length of tube.

v Velocity of a fluid.

v_B Velocity of an idealized Bingham plastic at radius r_f in a tube.

v_C Velocity of a fluid obeying the Casson equation at radius r_f in a tube.

v_N Velocity of a Newtonian fluid at radius r_f in a tube.

v_{pl} Velocity of a power-law fluid at radius r_f in a tube.

$\bar{v}_t$ Mean velocity of flow in a tube.

w_f Weight of fibrinogen per 100 ml of suspending fluid.

x Diameter of core of suspension in a tube.

y $\Omega/\bar{\tau}$.

α Longitudinal extension per unit of relaxed length.

β Lateral contraction per unit of relaxed length.

γ Displacement of a unit cube.

η Coefficient of viscosity of a fluid $= \tau/D$.

η_K Viscosity modulus of a Kelvin solid.

η_M Viscosity modulus of a Maxwell fluid.

η_a Apparent viscosity of a fluid.

η_o Viscosity of a suspending Newtonian fluid.

η_p Plastic viscosity of an idealized Bingham plastic.

η_r Relative viscosity of a suspension $= \eta_s/\eta_o$.

η_{ra} Apparent relative viscosity of a suspension, measured in a tube of radius R_i.

$\eta_{ra(min)}$ Minimum value of η_{ra}.

η_{rc} Viscosity of a suspension flowing in a core down a tube, relative to the viscosity of the suspending Newtonian fluid.

η_s Viscosity of a suspension.

ρ Density of a fluid.

σ Poisson's ratio $= \alpha/\beta$.

τ Tangential or shear stress.

$\bar{\tau}$ Arithmetic mean tangential stress in a co-axial cylinder viscometer.

τ_K Stress in a Kelvin solid at any instant.

τ_M Stress remaining in a Maxwell fluid after time t.

τ_e Extensive or tensional stress applied to a body.

τ_w Tangential stress in a fluid at a tube wall.

τ_y Yield stress of a Bingham plastic.

ψ Cone-plate viscometer angle (in radians).

Ω Angular velocity of the outer cylinder of a co-axial cylinder viscometer.

CHAPTER 1

RHEOLOGICAL CONCEPTS†

SUPPOSE that two smooth, parallel planes are introduced at unit distance apart into an infinitely large volume of a medium and that opposing forces are applied along the surfaces in order to displace them relative to each other. Consider a cube of the medium which is bounded on two sides by the planes and on the other four by the

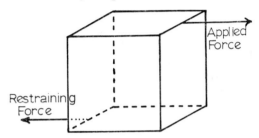

FIG. 1.1. Tangential forces on a cube of medium.

medium (Fig. 1.1). It will be assumed that no slip occurs at the interfaces between the planes and the medium and that the motion of the medium at the point of contact with the plane is the same as that of the plane itself.

The Solid State

If the cube of medium is of unit volume in terms of the dimensions being used, the force is being applied to opposite faces of the cube over unit area and is generally referred to as the *tangential* or *shear stress* τ. If the medium does not change its form when the tangential stress is applied it is termed a *rigid solid*. Normally, however, some deformation will occur. The medium may exert a restraining force

† Standard works dealing with rheology include Eirich (1956), Reiner (1960) and Fredrickson (1964).

on the displaced plane, and if the two planes return to their original positions when the stress is removed, the medium is called *elastic*. In general, the ratio of the stress applied to the *displacement* or *strain* achieved gives the *modulus of elasticity*; if the displacement is completely recovered when the stress is removed and the elasticity modulus has a constant value, the medium is termed *perfectly elastic* or *Hookean*. In the case of a tangential stress τ producing a displacement γ (Fig. 1.2) the *shear* or *rigidity modulus* is obtained. Many

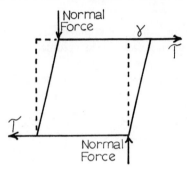

FIG. 1.2. Deformation of a solid cube by a tangential stress.

solids approximate closely to Hookean behaviour provided that the stress is small and is applied slowly, and that the displacement is small. A large stress may cause the solid to flow or to fracture, irreversibly disturbing the relative positions of the solid elements. If the stresses to which the unit cube are exposed are exactly as shown in Fig. 1.1 the cube will rotate in a clockwise direction until the applied stresses lie in the same plane. This rotation is prevented by the normal forces exerted by the parallel planes on the medium

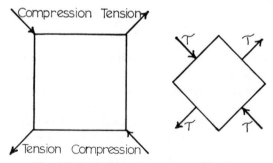

FIG. 1.3. Equivalent stresses on a solid cube.

as illustrated in Fig. 1.2. It can easily be shown that for small displacements the tangential stress is equivalent to a pair of tensional forces and a pair of compressive forces mutually perpendicular to each other and equivalent to normal stresses of τ acting on the faces of a cube of the material as in Fig. 1.3. Thus tangential forces are not essential for producing shear and it is quite usual to measure certain elastic moduli by applying compressive or tensional forces to a body.

If only tensional stresses are applied to a unit cube of material (Fig. 1.4) and they result in a small displacement or strain in the direction of the stress α, and a corresponding lateral contraction β,

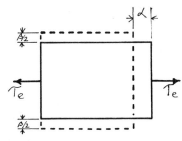

FIG. 1.4. Deformation of a solid cube by an elongating stress.

$$\text{Young's modulus } E = \frac{\tau_e}{\alpha}$$

and $$\text{Poisson's ratio } \sigma = \frac{\beta}{\alpha}$$

where τ_e = tensional stress applied to the cube.

Young's modulus can be obtained without difficulty from experiments on strips of biological tissue but Poisson's ratio is more difficult to measure. If no change in volume occurs under stress, however, $\sigma = 0\cdot5$ and this value is often assumed for the walls of blood vessels (Lawton, 1955) in the absence of more complete data. The value of the shear modulus then equals $\frac{1}{3}$ of the Young's modulus.

Elastic Tubes

If the pressure inside an elastic-walled tube of constant length and inside radius R_i (Fig. 1.5) is increased by an amount ΔP_w above the outer pressure so that the outer radius R_o increases by some

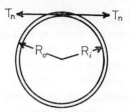

FIG. 1.5. Cross-section of an elastically walled tube.

value ΔR_o, Love (1927) has shown that the tangentially directed Young's modulus of the wall material E is given by

$$E = \frac{\Delta P_w}{\Delta R_o} \frac{2(1 - \sigma^2)R_i^2 R_o}{R_o^2 - R_i^2}.\qquad(1.1)$$

If the wall thickness is less than about one-tenth of the tube diameter and ΔP_w is small the tension in the wall T_n is given by the law of *Laplace*

$$T_n = \Delta P_w R_o$$

or

$$\tau_e = \frac{T_n}{R_o - R_i} = \frac{\Delta P_w R_o}{R_o - R_i}.$$

The displacement per unit length

$$a = \frac{\Delta R_o}{R_o}$$

so that

$$E = \frac{\tau_e}{a} = \frac{\Delta P_w R_o^2}{\Delta R_o(R_o - R_i)}.\qquad(1.2)$$

Both eqns. (1.1) and (1.2) have been used for determining the Young's modulus of blood vessels (Bergel, 1961a, b; Peterson, 1964). Other criteria, such as the volume distensibility $(\Delta V/\Delta P_w)V$ where ΔV is the change in volume of a length of blood vessel of volume V produced by a change ΔP_w in pressure have also been used but they have the disadvantage of being dependent upon both the elasticity of the wall and the geometry of the vessel so that direct comparisons become difficult to make.

The Fluid State

Referring again to Fig. 1.1, if no restraining forces have developed inside the medium when the motion of the moving plane ceases, the planes will remain in their new relative positions when the tangential stress is removed. A medium such as this, which is unable to sustain internal forces, is termed a *fluid*; it can be either a liquid or a gas.

For a fluid to be sheared continuously, a constant tangential stress must be applied to it and if the constant velocity achieved by the moving plane is directly proportional to the tangential stress applied, the fluid obeys Newton's law of proportionality between stress and velocity. Such a fluid is therefore termed *Newtonian*. The tangential stress which is required to maintain unit velocity difference between the two parallel faces of the cube of fluid situated unit distance apart is termed the *coefficient of viscosity* η. Thus, if in general a tangential stress τ produces a displacement D in unit time between planes situated unit distance apart,

$$\eta = \frac{\tau}{D}. \tag{1.3}$$

D is frequently termed the *rate of shear* or the *velocity gradient* and equals dy/dt or $\dot{\gamma}$ but it should be noted that "rate of shear" and "velocity gradient" are only synonymous when the lines of shear are straight and parallel. If C.G.S. units are employed, the viscosity is given in *poise*, a unit which is named after the French physician Poiseuille who was the first experimenter to make exact measurements of viscous resistance. Very many common fluids (such as water and air) are almost Newtonian in behaviour, the deviations being insignificantly small for most practical purposes. On the other hand, in theoretical fluid mechanics it is not unusual in some circumstances to ignore the viscosity of the fluid, which is then termed *inviscid*.

There are many practical fluids, particularly liquids, for which the velocity of the moving plane is not proportional to the applied stress and they are termed *non-Newtonian*. Such a fluid cannot possess a single, constant coefficient of viscosity, and values calculated from the ratio of the applied tangential stress to the rate of shear produced are called *apparent viscosities*. A plot of the tangential stress against the rate of shear produces the *flow curve* of the material and for a Newtonian fluid it consists of a straight line passing through the origin (Fig. 1.6).

Rheological Models

The concepts of solidity and fluidity are idealizations which describe the behaviour of real materials in certain limiting cases. In general the behaviour of a real material encompasses many intermediate properties which are summarized in Fig. 1.7.

A convenient way of visualizing the various types of behaviour of matter is by analogy to the behaviour of mechanical models.

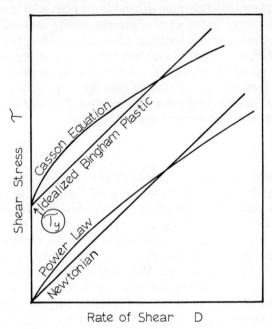

FIG. 1.6. Flow curves of various model materials.

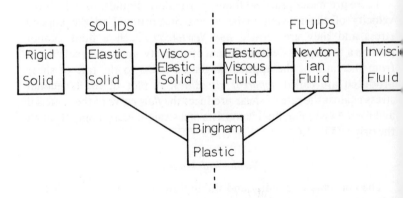

FIG. 1.7. Types of rheological materials.

Thus the model analogous to a viscous fluid is the dashpot assembly (Fig. 1.8). It has the property of being unable to support any stress and the rate of shearing is a direct function of the applied stress. In the case of a Newtonian fluid there would be direct proportionality

Force

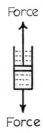

Force

FIG. 1.8. Mechanical model of a viscous fluid.

between the applied stress and the rate of shearing. For an inviscid fluid the liquid in the dashpot would have negligible viscosity.

The flow properties of many non-Newtonian fluids can be expressed by the so-called "power-law" formula, where the consistency parameter

$$K_{pl} = \frac{\tau}{D^s} \qquad (1.4)$$

where s = a constant. It should be noted that some authors use the reciprocal of s as the exponential parameter.

It is apparent that K_{pl} is only dimensionless in the case of $s = 1$, when it is equal to the viscosity. Otherwise K_{pl} depends both upon the nature of the material and on the dimensions in which τ and D are expressed. Suspensions of red cells often appear to behave as power-law fluids but although the relationship is useful for anticipating interpolated values and in calculating velocity profiles, there

Force

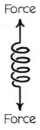

Force

FIG. 1.9. Mechanical model of an elastic solid.

is no evidence that it has any physical significance or can be interpreted in terms of the properties of the constituents of the fluid. The flow curve for a power-law fluid is shown in Fig. 1.6.

The mechanical model for the elastic solid is the spring (Fig. 1.9). In this case the extension is a function of the applied force and if it is removed the spring reverts immediately to its unstretched position. For a rigid solid the spring is so strong that no extension is possible, irrespective of the load applied.

The Maxwell elastico-viscous fluid is represented by a spring and a dashpot in series (Fig. 1.10). It is appropriate to call such a material

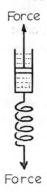

Force

Force

FIG. 1.10. Mechanical model of a Maxwell fluid.

a fluid because the application of any force, however small, will lead to continuous flow. On the other hand it exhibits *relaxation*. Suppose the model is subjected to a sudden extension which is then maintained. The initial extension is only in the spring which, as time proceeds, contracts and pulls out the dashpot cylinder thus maintaining the system at a constant elongation. When the spring has contracted to its equilibrium position relaxation is complete. If the applied force is released before the internal deformation has ceased, the spring is still under tension and the system recoils but not to its original configuration.

The stress τ_M, remaining at a time t after the application of a shear stress τ, is given by

$$\tau_M = \eta_M D + (\tau - \eta_M D)^{-(E_M/\eta_M)t}. \tag{1.5}$$

where η_M and E_M are the viscosity and elasticity moduli of the material respectively.

When flow ceases the rate of shear D becomes zero and the stress τ_M falls exponentially to zero. The possibility of blood behaving under certain circumstances as an elastico-viscous fluid is discussed in Chapter 6.

The Kelvin visco-elastic solid which is sometimes referred to as a Voigt body is represented by a spring and dashpot arranged in parallel (Fig. 1.11). It is a model of a solid because the maximum

Force

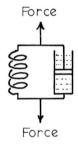

Force

FIG. 1.11. Mechanical model of a Kelvin solid.

extension which can be achieved is limited by the force applied and is independent of the time of application. The model exhibits the phenomenon of *creep*. If a constant force is applied, the extension gradually increases up to a maximum value determined by the magnitude of the applied force. The stress τ_K at any instant is given by

$$\tau_K = E_K\gamma + \eta_K D \qquad (1.6)$$

where E_K and η_K are the elasticity and viscosity moduli respectively. If the force is released the model will gradually recover its initial configuration. There is some evidence that the walls of the blood vessels and the surface membrane of red cells behave as visco-elastic solids.

Many practical materials combine elastic and viscous elements in such a way that they exhibit both relaxation and creep and it is not possible to express their properties in terms of springs and dashpots.

The model of a Bingham plastic is shown in Fig. 1.12. Friction between the sliding surfaces makes extension of the system impossible unless the applied force exceeds the frictional force. This force represents the *yield stress* of the material under shear. If the rate of extension of the system is exactly proportional to the applied stress which is in excess of the yield stress, the material is called an *idealized Bingham plastic*. It is very doubtful whether any known material behaves in this way, except to a crude approximation, but the con-

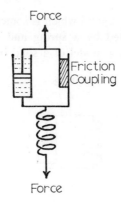

Force

Friction
Coupling

Force

FIG. 1.12. Mechanical model of a Bingham plastic.

cept is a simple and useful one and a typical curve is illustrated in Fig. 1.6. Two coefficients are required to classify an idealized Bingham plastic, the yield stress τ_y and the plastic viscosity η_p. They are connected by the equation

$$\eta_p = \frac{\tau - \tau_y}{D}. \tag{1.7}$$

Practical materials may also possess a modulus of elasticity which is operative below the yield stress but this is ignored in most cases. It will be observed that if flow measurements are made at high rates of shear $\tau \gg \tau_y$ and the apparent viscosity of the suspension τ/D tends asymptotically towards the plastic viscosity $(\tau - \tau_y)/D$.

A modification to the equation for an idealized Bingham plastic has been proposed by Casson (1959). If K_C is a measure of the consistency of the material

$$K_C = \frac{\sqrt{\tau} - \sqrt{\tau_y}}{\sqrt{D}}. \tag{1.8}$$

For high rates of shear or a low yield stress

$$K_C \to \sqrt{\left(\frac{\tau}{D}\right)} \to \sqrt{\eta}.$$

Whole blood has been shown by some experimenters to follow the Casson equation but although attempts have been made to give it a physical basis the equation should still be considered as empirical. A typical flow curve for a Casson-equation plastic is included in Fig. 1.6.

In some cases the flow properties of a material depend upon its immediate history. For example, the apparent viscosity of a bentonite suspension generally decreases after it has been stirred vigorously. This dependence of flow properties upon time is termed *thixotropy*. It is not a phenomenon which has been widely reported in connection with the vascular system although this may be because few specific attempts have been made to detect it. The continuous change in the flow properties of blood which occurs on its removal from a living body is caused by the operation of the normal clotting mechanisms; this does not make blood thixotropic however, because the changes which occur are irreversible.

Solutions and Suspensions

Important changes are observed in the flow properties of Newtonian liquids when particles or large molecules are dispersed in them. These must be appreciated before the behaviour of plasma or suspensions of red cells can be understood.

Consider the effect of introducing discrete particulate matter into a unit cube of Newtonian fluid which is being sheared between

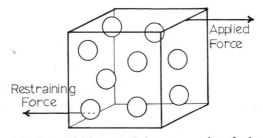

Fig. 1.13. Tangential force applied to a suspension of spheres.

parallel faces (Fig. 1.13). The bodies replace some of the liquid in the original cube of suspending medium so that the mean rate at which the remainder of the liquid is sheared by a given velocity difference between the moving planes is greater than if the particulate matter were absent. Thus the resistance of the suspension to flow is increased; the question of whether the mixture will exhibit Newtonian properties or not depends upon the characteristics and concentration of the dispersed matter.

Rigid Particles

Spheres. A suspension of rigid, non-interacting, non-settling spheres at concentrations so low that mechanical interference between them can be ignored is Newtonian and the determination of its viscosity becomes a fluid dynamic problem. Einstein (1906) first solved it satisfactorily and found that the viscosity of the suspension η_s was related to the viscosity of the suspending liquid η_o by the equation

$$\eta_s = \eta_o(1 + 2 \cdot 5c)$$

where c is the volume of particles contained in a unit volume of suspension and is frequently termed the solids volume concentration. Volume concentration is generally expressed as a percentage of the total volume of suspension rather than as a fraction of it and this convention will be followed here.

Often interest is focused on the influence of the added particles on the viscosity level and it is simpler to consider the viscosity of the suspension relative to that of the suspending liquid. The *relative viscosity* η_r† is given by

$$\eta_r = \frac{\eta_s}{\eta_0} = 1 + 2 \cdot 5c.$$

The *specific viscosity* is also used and is defined as

$$\eta_r - 1 = 2 \cdot 5c, \text{ for spheres.}$$

Other workers, particularly those working with low concentrations of polymers, prefer the *intrinsic viscosity* which is defined as

$$\frac{\eta_r - 1}{c} = 2 \cdot 5, \text{ for spheres.} \tag{1.9}$$

If the concentration of rigid spheres is increased above about 1 per cent, mutual interference occurs between them and additional

† It is important to note that in physiology the relative viscosity is often defined as the viscosity of a fluid relative to water. This differs from the definition used here and elsewhere in the book.

liquid is immobilized during collisions. Thus the viscosity rises faster with concentration than predicted by Einstein's equation. A useful modification of his equation by Oliver *et al.* (1953) which is valid up to a volume concentration of about 30 per cent and has been given a theoretical basis by Sadron (1953) and Maude (1960) is

$$\eta_r = \frac{1}{1 - 2 \cdot 5c} = 1 + 2 \cdot 5c + 6 \cdot 25c^2 + \ldots$$

It is important to note that the size of the spheres does not influence the viscosity of the suspension if, of course, they are large compared with the size of the molecules of the suspending liquid. Moreover, the relative, specific and intrinsic viscosities of spheres are all independent of the viscosity of the suspending liquid and give a measure of the magnitude of the interacting forces which exist in the suspension. Above a concentration of about 40 per cent there is some evidence of the development of non-Newtonian behaviour in suspensions of spheres (Rutgers, 1962) and the analysis of the system becomes extremely difficult.

It has long been recognized that when a closely packed mass of static grains is sheared there is a tendency for it to expand at right-angles to the direction of shear. This is termed *dilation* and it can only be resisted by the application of a compressive stress during shear. Bagnold (1954) showed that a similar effect can be detected in suspensions of rigid spheres at volume concentrations as low as 13 per cent. Where the shear rate was low and the fluid was very viscous

$$\text{Dispersive pressure} = 0 \cdot 65 \, D\eta_0 \, \frac{\left(c_0/c\right)^{\frac{1}{3}} \left[2 \left(c_0/c\right)^{\frac{1}{3}} - 1\right]}{\left[\left(c_0/c\right)^{\frac{1}{3}} - 1\right]^2} \quad (1.10)$$

where c_0 is the maximum possible static volume concentration of particles (0·74 for spheres). It should be noted that the dispersive pressure is of different origin, and generally of much smaller magnitude, than the *normal force* which develops at right-angles to the direction of shear during the flow of solutions of some long-chain molecules.

Other Shapes. If the particles are not spherical the mechanism of interaction becomes very complicated even at low concentrations. For example, a single rigid ellipsoid rotates in a series of complex but predictable orbits in a shearing fluid unless its axis of symmetry happens to lie parallel to the shearing plane and perpendicular to the direction of the tangential stress when simple rotation takes place (Fig. 1.14). The motion of, and interaction between, particles

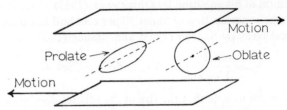

FIG. 1.14. Orientations of ellipsoids in a shearing fluid which give simple rotation.

has been extensively studied by Mason and his collaborators (Goldsmith *et al.*, 1967). The usual result of replacing spheres by smooth, rigid, randomly oriented particles of other shapes is to increase the interaction forces at the same concentration and raise the relative viscosity. Thus at low concentrations

$$\eta_r = 1 + K_1 c \tag{1.11}$$

where K_1 is greater than $2 \cdot 5$ and increases with increasing asymmetry of the particles.

The shearing of a dilute suspension of identical, geometrically shaped, rigid particles such as ellipsoids, rods or discs which are initially randomly oriented tends to rearrange them so that they spend the majority of their time with their long axis roughly parallel to the plane of shear, flipping over from time to time according to the mechanism proposed by Jeffrey (1922) and confirmed by Mason and his co-workers (Goldsmith *et al.*, 1967). The viscosity of the suspension is independent of the rate of shear but as both theoretical and experimental determinations of its value are difficult to make, the figures for intrinsic viscosity [eqn. (1.9)] which are quoted in Table 1.1 should be considered as only approximate.

If the particles are very small, Brownian movement influences their final orientation under shear by trying to maintain the random distribution of their axes which they possessed when the suspension or solution was not under shear. In this case the viscosity decreases with increasing rate of shear (because the orientation of the particles increases) until it finally reaches the same value as for larger particles of the same shape (Sadron, 1953). Typical maximum values at low rates of shear are included in Table 1.1. Brownian movement is

TABLE 1.1

Intrinsic viscosity of suspensions of rigid bodies

Shape	Aspect ratio	Intrinsic viscosity	
		No Brownian motion	With Brownian motion (maximum value)
Spheres	—	2·5	2·5
Rods	20	5·0[1]	30[2]
Ellipsoids (prolate)	20	12[3]	38[3]
Rods	50	10[1]	100[2]
Ellipsoids (prolate)	50	47[3]	177[3]
Ellipsoids (oblate)	0·2	3·0[3]	4·7[4]
Flexible discs	0·18	1·4[5]	—

[1] Experiments of Nawab *et al.* (1958).
[2] Experiments reported by Sadron (1953).
[3] Theory of Scheraga (1955).
[4] Theory of Simha (1940).
[5] Experiments of Müller (1936) at low flow velocities in tubes.

only important for particles of less than about 1 μ in size so that although it should affect the orientation of the protein molecules in blood plasma it is doubtful whether red cells would be noticeably influenced by it.

As the concentration of the dispersed phase is raised, the number of interactions between particles increases rapidly, and the viscosity rises steeply. Reliable quantitative data applicable to blood are not at present available although some experimental results on rubber discs flowing in tubes have been reported by Müller (1936).

Flexible Particles

Most of the work on flexible particles has been carried out with the object of explaining the flow behaviour of solutions of long-chain molecules. These are represented as curled, branched, elastic threads of great length (compared to their width) and are not particularly representative of any of the constituents of normal blood. Nevertheless, it is likely that the flexibility of red cells has an important bearing on the flow behaviour of blood and particularly on its non-Newtonian properties. At very low rates of shear it might be expected that the deformation of the cells would be small enough for them to behave as rigid bodies. At higher shear rates, however, deformation of the cells could be appreciable but the question of whether this would increase or reduce the viscosity is impossible to answer without detailed information on the extent to which the type and number of interactions are affected.

Bingham plastic behaviour is frequently exhibited by aggregated or flocculated suspensions in which the concentration of particles is sufficiently great for a continuous structure to form on standing. Under the influence of small stresses the structure may deform elastically, so that flow only commences when the applied stress is sufficiently large to break the inter-particle bonds (Roscoe, 1953; Michaels *et al.*, 1962; Obiakor *et al.*, 1964). For rigid particles of a given shape, the plastic viscosity is primarily dependent upon the concentration of particles present, and the yield stress upon a combination of the particle concentration and the inter-particle forces. In general it has been shown that the yield stress is given by

$$\tau_y = K_2(c - c_{min})^3 \qquad (1.12)$$

where K_2 = a constant, and c_{min} = minimum volume concentration at which a structure forms (Michaels *et al.*, 1962). A similar type of equation has been applied to blood (Merrill *et al.*, 1964).

CHAPTER 2

THE CIRCULATING SYSTEM†

THE overall organization of the cardiovascular system is illustrated diagrammatically in Fig. 2.1. The chambers of the right and left side of the heart are connected through two parallel vascular beds: the systemic (or peripheral) and the pulmonary circulation. The left ventricle pumps oxygenated blood into the aorta, which is a long, arch-shaped vessel, from which smaller arteries and arterioles distribute it into a number of parallel vascular beds which form the systemic circulation. As the blood passes through the capillary network of the various organ systems of the body it exchanges oxygen, carbon dioxide, foodstuffs, metabolites and water with the tissue cells. After this exchange across the capillary membrane, the blood leaves the capillaries with a reduced oxygen saturation, an increased content of metabolites and carbon dioxide and a decreased pH. It is collected by the venules in the venous system and flows back through the venae cavae to the right atrium, from which it passes to the right ventricle. The right ventricle pumps the blood through the pulmonary arteries into the pulmonary capillaries, where the exchange of oxygen and carbon dioxide with the atmosphere takes place. The re-oxygenated blood flows through the pulmonary venous system into the left atrium and the left ventricle from where it is returned to the aorta.

The arterioles, capillaries and venules form the microcirculation although the exact points at which it merges into the arterial or the venous systems of tissue is by no means clear. The reason is that in the areas where the different kinds of vessels join each other they often fail to exhibit differences for appreciable distances (Bloch, 1966b). On the other hand, the vessels can be defined readily if the

---

† Standard works covering various parts of the field are too numerous to list here but references to authors who deal with specific topics are included in the text.

definition is derived from data secured from the midportion of their total length.

The vascular system consists of a huge and complicated network of elastic, or visco-elastic, tubes. Through continuous dichotomous branching, the single tract from the heart ultimately splits into more than 100 million channels the total cross-section of which is several hundred times as large as that of the aorta. The problem of extra-polating present hydrodynamic and rheological methods of analysis

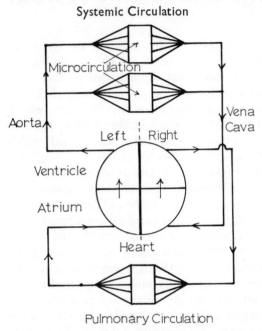

Fig. 2.1. Diagrammatic representation of the circulation.

to this intricate architecture is obviously very great but a primary requirement is detailed information regarding the physical properties of the various vessels and of the blood which flows through them. This is presented, so far as it is available, in the present chapter. The functional characteristics of the heart will not be considered because its structure and the dynamics of its operation, which have been ex-tensively studied and documented (Guyton, 1963), are outside the scope of the present work. The problems associated with the flow of blood in specific organs are also ignored but it may be noted that very little information is available of the extent to which their operation is influenced by the flow properties of the blood.

Blood Vessels

Arteries

The arteries are often divided into two functional categories; elastic types, such as the aorta, which are the main transporting vessels for the blood, and muscular types which distribute the blood to the capillary beds (Burton, 1962; Tuttle et al., 1965). There are three major wall constituents—elastin, collagen and smooth muscle —and typical figures for their Young's moduli are given in Table 2.1.

TABLE 2.1

Young's modulus of biological materials

Material	Young's modulus (dyne/cm^2)
Collagen	10^8–10^9 [1]
Elastin	3–6×10^6 [1, 2, 3]
Smooth muscle	10^5–10^7 [1, 2, 4]
Soft vulcanized rubber	15–50×10^6 [5]
Polyethylene	3×10^9

[1] Burton (1954).   [4] Hinke et al. (1962).
[2] Bergel (1964, 1966). [5] Kaye et al. (1959).
[3] Carton et al. (1962).

Of the three the properties of smooth muscle are the most difficult to measure and the resulting values are the least reliable because its properties alter as its activity changes (Bergel, 1964). It should be noted that the Young's modulus of collagen is appreciably greater than that of the other constituents and rises as it is extended (Bergel, 1966).

In elastic arteries, smooth muscle in amounts that increase toward the periphery lies obliquely between adjacent elastic laminae which may number up to 50 in the aorta (Bergel, 1966). In any layer the muscle cells are arranged in parallel array to form a helix but successive layers are oriented in different directions so that the forces are complexly distributed (Fig. 2.2). Collagen fibres are plentiful within the wall, forming a loose unattached basketwork around the other structures (Pease, 1962; Bergel, 1964). The smaller distributing arteries differ histologically from the larger transporting arteries in having a lower proportion of elastic connective tissue in their walls and more collagen fibres (Fig. 2.2) but there is no sharp demarcation between the types. The contraction of muscle cells to a rounder shape stiffens the walls of muscular arteries whereas in elastic arteries it tends to thicken the wall, reducing the effective diameter of the vessel but not necessarily increasing its stiffness (Bergel, 1966). In every case the innermost surface of the wall is lined with a layer of cells, termed the endothelium which is believed to be hydrophilic in healthy living animals (Burton, 1964; Tuttle et al., 1965) although

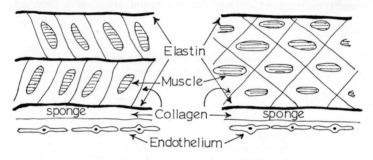

FIG. 2.2. Typical structure of artery walls (after Bergel, 1966).

this has been questioned (Copley et al., 1964). The high pressures developed by the blood in the arterial system lead to compression of the endothelium and it possesses a very smooth surface of characteristically thin flat hexagons whose long axes are aligned with the direction of flow (Rodbard, 1962).

The cross-sections of arteries are normally circular but some branches have been found to be elliptic (Caro et al., 1966), a value of $1\cdot91 \pm 0\cdot16$ being reported for the aspect ratio of the right pulmonary artery (Attinger, 1964b). The ratio of the wall thickness to the vessel radius has been measured on numbers of occasions giving values varying from $0\cdot07$ to $0\cdot13$ (Peterson, 1964). Although it is generally believed that the wall thickness increases relative to the vessel radius as the radius of the vessel diminishes (Burton, 1965), other evidence is that in the arterial system the ratio is fairly constant at $0\cdot1$–$0\cdot16$ (McDonald 1960b). Thus measurements of

Young's modulus in the tangential direction in the wall of an artery can be made with good reliability in most cases by measuring the change in radius with change in pressure and using eqn. 1.2 which applies for ratios of wall thickness to vessel diameter of less than about $0 \cdot 1$, although some corrections may be required if the vessels are elliptic in cross-section (Attinger, 1964b). The arteries appear to be well tethered in the surrounding tissue so that longitudinal displacements under the pulsating action of the blood are probably very small (Patel et al., 1964) but an exception may be found in the case of the pulmonary artery and the aorta which can move in sympathy with the heart to which they are attached.

The heterogeneity of the wall structure makes its stress–strain characteristics rather complex, the static Young's modulus increasing with the extension. For instance, Evans et al., (1962) found that the cross-section of a dog aorta changed linearly with pressure. In other words $\Delta R_o / \Delta P_w \propto 1/R_o$ and not $\propto R_o^2$ as required by eqn. 1.2 for a material of constant Young's modulus. The reason for this behaviour cannot be found in the properties of the individual wall constituents. The function of the smooth muscle is to control the diameters of the arteries by contracting or expanding under physiological control and it probably makes only a minor alteration to their elastic properties (McDonald, 1960b). Elastin and collagen alone approximate quite closely to Hookean behaviour but they are so disposed in the artery wall that the elastin first comes under tension at small extensions (see Fig. 2.2). It is believed that as the stress is raised, more and more of the high elastic-modulus collagen fibres reach their unstretched length and add their contributions to the tension in the wall (Roach et al., 1957; Burton, 1965). Thus the Young's modulus of excised dog artery ranges from 6 to 8×10^6 dyne/cm² at the stresses normally applying in the arterial system to 10^6 dyne/cm² at stresses of one-fifth normal when the elastin has a corrugated appearance (McDonald, 1960b; Bergel, 1966).

One important physiological consequence of the change in elastic modulus with the applied stress should be mentioned. It will be recalled from eqn. (1.2) that

$$\text{Young's modulus } E = \frac{\tau_e}{\Delta R_o / R_o}$$

or

$$\frac{\Delta R_o}{R_o} = \frac{\tau_e}{E}.$$

The normal pulsations of the heart, which produce a fluctuation of about $\pm$ 20 per cent in the mean pressure difference across the arterial wall, therefore lead to a similar variation in the tensional stress τ_e in the wall from the Laplace equation (see p. 4). But the elastic modulus E is also altered sufficiently for the radius of the vessel to vary by less than 5 per cent (McDonald, 1960b; Peterson, 1962; Attinger, 1967) instead of the anticipated 30 or 40 per cent change. Indirect evidence from the velocity of the pulse wave and the change in structure of the walls suggests that the Young's modulus should increase progressively with the distance of the artery from the heart (McDonald, 1960b) but direct measurements and deductions from pulse velocity (Hinke *et al.*, 1962; Spencer *et al.*, 1963) do not always confirm this.

The percentage elongation which aorta walls can undergo before rupture is about 50 per cent and only about one-third of the value for rubber (Dintenfass, 1963a). With age the Young's modulus of the arteries increases but as the ratio of wall thickness to vessel radius also decreases, the volume distensibility relationship (see p. 4) may remain almost constant (Peterson, 1964). This is one of the reasons why it is an unsatisfactory index of the stress–strain characteristics of arteries.

The walls also exhibit visco-elastic properties, the major determinant of the viscous component lying in the smooth muscle (Bergel, 1966; Apter *et al.*, 1966). Peterson (1964) reported that the mechanical properties of the aorta and its branches in dogs were equivalent to those of a Kelvin solid, obeying eqn. (1.6). Models using more complex arrays of elastic and viscous elements have also been proposed (Ranke, 1934; Apter, 1964) leading to the possibility of the walls exhibiting both creep and relaxation (Peterson, 1962). No simple model accounts fully for their behaviour, particularly under the influence of cyclic forces and they are probably best described by the simplest model with the addition of a frequency-dependent term (Hardung, 1962). Measurements made in the physiological range of frequencies (less than 20 c/s) show that the dynamic elastic modulus EK is greater than the static E by a ratio which depends upon the position of the artery in the body and ranges from $1\cdot05$ for the thoracic aorta to $1\cdot6$ for the carotid artery of dogs (Bergel, 1961b). Above about 1 or 2 c/s the dynamic modulus remains substantially constant (Bergel, 1964; McDonald *et al.*, 1967), unlike other visco-elastic materials which become stiffer with increasing frequency.

The corresponding viscosity has been estimated as about 10^4 poise (Peterson, 1962), increasing with the degree of extension. These general conclusions can probably be applied to a variety of mammals because there is evidence that the elastic properties of the main human arteries do not differ greatly from those of the dog (Patel et al., 1964).

All arteries taper slightly along their length. Where bifurcations of blood-distributing vessels occur the diameters of the secondary arteries are usually approximately equal in diameter and 10–20 per cent smaller than that of the feed vessel (McDonald, 1960b; Caro et al., 1966).

Arterioles

The arterioles provide the greatest and the most variable resistance to blood flow because they are relatively narrow and contain an abundance of muscle in their walls (Fig. 2.3), (Rhodin, 1962; Wiederhielm, 1965). Their diameters are actively controlled by the state of contraction of this smooth muscle and can alter from complete closure to dilation up to two (Jeffords et al., 1956) or four times the normal diameter (Merrill et al., 1961), which ranges from 15 to 500 μ according to Merrill et al. (1961) although other investigators have set an upper limit which is much smaller than this (Maggio, 1965; Sobin, 1966). The factors which influence arteriole muscle contractions are manifold and will not be considered here but they can be divided into nervous, chemical and physical (Haddy, 1962). *In vivo* experiments show that the static elastic modulus of relaxed arterioles is very similar to, or a little less than, that of muscular arteries. It rises rapidly as the stress is in-

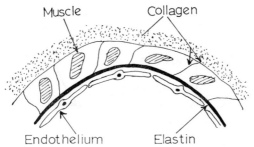

FIG. 2.3. Structure of the arteriole wall in the frog mesentery (after Wiederhielm, 1965).

creased so that with strains as low as 0.05 at least 80 per cent of the stress is taken by the collagen in the wall (Wiederhielm, 1964, 1965). At strains exceeding 0.25 the modulus increases particularly quickly, reaching a value of 45×10^6 dyne/cm² for a strain of 0.31 (Wiederhielm, 1964). Although the viscosity modulus of the wall η_K is also strongly dependent upon the strain and rises linearly with it, it is also influenced by the activity of the muscle cells. In an arteriole actively constricted by the muscle cells to its relaxed size the viscosity modulus has been reported to be 40 times higher than in a relaxed arteriole, while at wall stresses of 8×10^6 dyne/cm² values for the modulus of viscosity of 3.6×10^9 poise have been observed (Wiederhielm, 1964).

The arterioles are lined internally with endothelial cells which play an insignificant part in their rheology. They taper slightly along their length; for example, the mesenteric arterioles of mice and frogs have a taper angle varying from $0°\ 5'$ to $2°\ 17'$ (Jeffords et al., 1956). It has been claimed that the narrowest portion in the vascular system is just before the arterioles join the capillaries (Saunders et al., 1954) but it is possible that some capillaries are even narrower and are capable of complete closure (Maggio, 1965).

Capillaries

Capillaries are the vascular channels in which exchange of materials between blood and tissue, and vice versa, primarily occurs. They are generally untapered and appear in mammals as tubes some $3–15\ \mu$ in diameter formed by a single layer of flat endothelial cells, possibly held together by an intercellular cement but without reinforcement, or elastin or collagen support (Krogh, 1959; Luft, 1964) (Fig. 2.4). The layer of cells is enclosed by a "basement membrane" which plays an important part in transcapillary molecular exchange

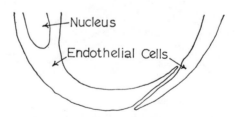

FIG. 2.4. Typical structure of a capillary wall (after Fawcett, 1959).

(Maggio, 1965). One or more cells seem to constitute the wall at a given point of the vessel, longitudinal sections showing a mosaic-like organization of rhomboid or polygonal endothelial cells, arranged in a spiral form (Mayerson, 1962). The thickness of the walls is 2–3 μ at the level of the maximum diameter of the nucleus and 300 Å near the edge of the cell where it overlaps its neighbour. Molecules up to the size of inulin, equivalent to a molecular weight of 5200 and a diameter of about 30 Å are able to pass easily through the walls, probably by diffusion (Maggio, 1965), and most easily towards the venous end (Intaglietta, 1967). There is also a second, or large-pore system behaving as a much smaller population of channels some 350 Å in diameter (Landis *et al.*, 1963). The surface exposed to the

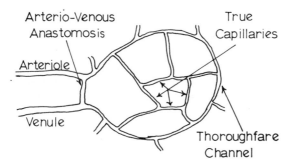

FIG. 2.5. Diagrammatic representation of the microcirculation (Sphincters and valves have been omitted for clarity).

blood is irregular, showing tiny pseudopod-like or fringe-like structures and it may be coated internally with a very thin layer of proteinaceous material—possibly fibrin (Copley, 1960)—although electron microscopy has not so far confirmed its presence (Fawcett, 1959). The flow velocity is, on average, less than 0·1 cm/sec and in many animals it is controlled by a sphincter, or valve, at the entrance.

Terminal vascular beds differ greatly in different regions of the microcirculation (Sobin, 1966) but are of fantastic complexity (Berman, 1964; Burton, 1965; Fulton *et al.*, 1967). Frequently the capillaries originate from the subdivision of precapillary channels which in turn diverge from a thoroughfare channel (Zweifach *et al.*, 1956) connecting a terminal arteriole with a collecting venule (Fig. 2.5) so that the branching network may be equipped with a variety of feeds and drains (Paterson *et al.*, 1967). Thoroughfare channels are characterized by a very sparsely distributed muscle coat only one cell thick and flow from them into the capillary network is often controlled by precapillary sphincters (Maggio, 1965). The angles of branching of capillaries differ in various organs and in different species. Thus in the lung and liver they radiate circumferentially at right-angles to the axis of the supplying vessels whereas in the mesentery they radiate at less acute angles of 30° to 45° (Bloch, 1963). A feature of many vascular beds is the existence of direct connections between terminal arteries and veins, or arterio-venous anastomoses (or shunts), which short-circuit the capillary systems (Burton, 1965). They are thick-walled vessels generally closed during normal tissue metabolism (Bloch, 1966b) and structurally more comparable with arterioles than capillaries (Buck, 1963).

Venules

These vessels consist of a single layer of endothelial cells adhering to a thin layer of collagen connective tissue which forms the outer wall. Smooth muscle cells are generally absent in the smallest venules (Burton, 1954) but are present in the larger ones (Moreci *et al.*, 1962). The endothelial cells are more rounded than in the arterial system (Rodbard, 1962) and the diameters of the vessels, which increase slightly but continuously along their length, range from 10 to 140 μ (Guyton, 1961). The greatest cross-sectional area of flow, and thus the lowest mean velocity of flow, is often found in this part of the circulation (Fulton *et al.*, 1967).

Veins

The structure of the walls of veins is basically similar to that of arteries, consisting of layers of muscle and elastic fibres bound with collagen connective tissue and lined with endothelial cells. The main differences are that they contain less muscle and elastic tissue than artery walls (Kirk, 1962; Moreci *et al.*, 1962) which raises the static elastic modulus two- to fourfold (Attinger, 1967). But the walls are also much thinner, so that the changes in radius occurring over the normal physiological range are more than twice those of arteries. Veins are generally non-rigid and unable to maintain their shape if the internal pressure is less than that of the surrounding tissue. Their internal diameter is normally greater than that of the corresponding artery and in man ranges from 140 μ for the smallest veins to about 2 cm for the venae cavae which feed into the right atrium of the heart.

They provide the main variable blood reservoir for the living body and a system of valves within the vessels is operative in order to prevent back flow in the extremities of erect animals (Greenfield, 1962).

In general, the behaviour of circulation tissue at any instant depends upon a variety of intrinsic and extrinsic factors (Clark et al., 1965). Intrinsic factors include the stress relaxation time constants, the potential for stress recovery, the combined elastic and viscous moduli, the prevailing level of smooth muscle tone, the effects of "tethering" and the mass loading by surrounding structures. Extrinsic factors include the time characteristics of the loading and the immediate previous stress history of the tissue.

Blood

The major task of the blood is to supply oxygen to the living tissue and return carbon dioxide to the lungs. In addition it is responsible for collecting food from the gastrointestinal tract, eliminating non-gaseous metabolites in the kidneys, neutralizing foreign biological agents which enter the system and dissipating heat through various surfaces (Attinger, 1964b).

Whole blood consists of a suspension of formed elements including red cells (or erythrocytes), white cells (or leucocytes), and platelets in a saline solution of three major types of protein—fibrinogen, globulin and albumin. This continuous suspending medium is termed *plasma*.

Formed Elements

Red Cells. The red cells dominate the particulate matter in blood, occupying on the average about 40–45 per cent by volume of the whole blood. The percentage of red cells is normally given in terms of *haematocrit*. This is the volume percentage of red cells and entrained plasma obtained by allowing the cells to settle out, generally after centrifuging from an initial volume of whole blood prevented from clotting by the addition of anticoagulants. The centrifuged red cells generally contain about 1–2 per cent of trapped plasma so that the haematocrit is normally a little greater than the volume concentration of red cells (Ponder, 1966) but the two terms will be used synonymously. The major function of the red cells is to transport oxygen to the living tissues. The haemoglobin which carries out this duty is exclusively associated with the red cells, each 100 ml of whole blood containing about 15 g of haemoglobin which is able to transport 20 ml of oxygen, when measured at 37°C and a pressure of 760 mm of mercury saturated with water (Merrill *et al.*, 1961). Each cell consists of a fine flexible membrane, possibly mounted on a supporting network (Lehmann *et al.*, 1961), surrounding the haemoglobin.

The cells have a density of about 1·08 g/ml and their shape is generally that of a biconcave discoid (Fig. 2.6). They begin life

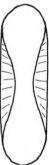

FIG. 2.6. Cross-section of a red blood cell.

complete with nucleus, mitochondria and microsomes but, in the case of mammals, later shed the nucleus (Bishop, 1964). Non-mammalian cells normally maintain the nucleus and mitochondria and may take the form of oval, rather than circular discoids. Immature cells (or reticulocytes) are larger and less dense than mature cells but normally only constitute about 1 per cent of the total red cells (Britton, 1963). Red cells become mechanically more fragile with age (Danon, 1967) and sometimes it is believed that the shrinkage which occurs when they mature proceeds continuously during their whole life (Bishop, 1964). The largest cells are found in tailed amphibia—for example those of the amphiuma are 70–80 μ long, 30 μ wide and 20 μ thick (Ponder, 1948) but mammalian cells are the smallest of any animal group. Typical dimensions are shown in Table 2.2 although the absolute values depend to some extent on the method of preparing the blood sample as illustrated in Table 2.3. Moreover,

TABLE 2.2

Size and shape of red cells

Mammal	Diameter (μ)		Thickness (μ)		Volume (μ^3)	$\dfrac{\text{Diameter}}{\text{Thickness}}$
	(1)	(2)	(1)	(2)	(1)	
Man	7·8	7·8	2·06	1·84	88	3·8–4·2
Dog	7·2	7·2	1·95	1·70	69	3·7–4·2
Rabbit	6·6	6·6	2·15	1·84	63	3·1–3·6
Cat	5·6	5·6	2·10	1·75	43	2·7–3·2
Goat	—	4·0	—	1·95	25	2·1

[1] Emmons (1927). Quoted by Lehmann et al. (1961).
[2] Haden (1934). Quoted by Britton (1963).

TABLE 2.3

Influence of method of preparation on red cell dimensions

Mammal	Diameter (μ)	Thickness (μ)		Volume (μ^3)	Method
		Max.	Min.		
Man	8·5	2·4	1·0	87	Wet [1]
Man	8·4	1·6		90	Wet [2]
Man	7·8	2·06		88	Unspecified [3]
Man	7·2	—		—	Stained film [4]
Rabbit	7·3	1·7	1·0	57	Wet [1]
Rabbit	6·6	1·84		63	Unspecified [3]

[1] Ponder (1948).
[2] Crosby (1952). Quoted by Britton (1963).
[3] Haden (1934). Quoted by Britton (1963).
[4] Price-Jones (1933). Quoted by Britton (1963).

the cells in any animal are never of identical size and typical ranges are given in Table 2.4.

It has been suggested that the cell size is related to the diameter of the capillaries (Lehmann et al., 1961) or the body-weight (Dunaway et al., 1965) of the particular animal and Table 2.2. shows that although the diameter varies a little from mammal to mammal the thickness is practically constant. This has been considered to have physiological significance (Lehmann et al., 1961). The question of the extent to which the unique shape and elastic properties of the red cells

TABLE 2.4

Size range of human red cells

Investigator	Range	Preparation method
Ponder (1948) Price-Jones (1933)[1]	67% between 8–9 μ 68% between $6 \cdot 75$–$7 \cdot 65$ μ	Wet Stained film

[1] Quoted by Britton (1963).

are optimal for the task of oxygen transport in living bodies is a complex one with many facets, some of which will be considered in later chapters.

Human red cells are in osmotic equilibrium with plasma which has an osmotic pressure corresponding to that of an aqueous solution containing $0 \cdot 85$–$0 \cdot 90$ per cent sodium chloride. If they are placed in solutions of lower concentration they swell to spheres, releasing haemoglobin through the membrane (Ponder, 1948). The volume of sphered human cells is between $1 \cdot 60$ times and twice that of the isotonic volume (Ponder, 1948; Katchalsky *et al.*, 1960, Rand *et al.*, 1963); approximately one half of the cells are affected in a $0 \cdot 45$ per cent solution and the action is completed when the concentration falls to $0 \cdot 30$ per cent. If osmosis in hypotonic solutions is allowed to swell the cells and haemolysis eliminates the haemoglobin, a ghost is formed when the cell is put back in an isotonic solution. This has the same shape as the original cell (Katchalsky *et al.*, 1960), although the original thickness may not be quite regained (Ponder, 1948) suggesting that the membrane and not the internal constituents of the cell determines its form. The membrane keeps most of its original properties after haemolysis (Van Deenan *et al.*, 1964) and even drastic changes in the surface charge such as follow treatment with neuraminidase or proteolytic enzymes do not destroy the biconcave discoid form (Seaman *et al.*, 1963).

Membrane Structure. The membrane accounts for only some 3 per cent of the mass of the human red cell (Burton, 1965). Its thickness has been measured by various indirect methods and appears to be between 60 (Katchalsky *et al.*, 1960) and 200 Å (Ponder, 1948; Burton, 1965). It is almost impermeable to cations but very permeable to anions, the flow apparently being through a pore-like surface structure whose openings are equivalent to the size of a sodium or potassium molecule (Passow, 1964), Paganelli and Soloman suggesting a diameter of 7 Å for the pores (Katchalsky et al., 1960). Moskowitz and Calvin visualized the membrane as composed of long fibrillar molecules arranged so that the fibrils lay side by side parallel to the cell surface and joined together by lipids (Pennell, 1964) but many other models have been suggested (Danielli, 1958; Katchalsky et al., 1960; Dintenfass, 1962; Van Deenan et al., 1964). It is probable that the total lipid content of the cell lies in the membrane although the haemoglobin may, in part, also be bound to it (Pennell, 1964). Striking differences have been found in the lipid characteristics of red cells from different species which suggests that membrane properties may vary considerably from animal to animal (Van Deenan et al., 1964).

By micromanipulative methods Rand et al. (1964b) showed that the membrane of human cells could suffer great bending strains reversibly but was drastically changed by tangential stresses. The stiffness was equivalent to about $0 \cdot 02$ dyne/cm and the resistance to deformation, which was the same at the rim as in the concavity, was unaltered after the cell's shape changed to that of a sphere by osmosis. It may also exhibit visco-elastic properties corresponding to a Kelvin solid [eqn. (1.6)]. Katchalsky et al. (1960) calculated the elastic modulus to be about $2 \cdot 4 \times 10^7$ dyne/cm^2 and the viscosity modulus 10^8 poise, characterizing the membrane as fairly rigid. On the other hand, Dintenfass (1964a) has suggested that the rheological behaviour of blood is explicable only in terms of a two-phase red cell membrane structure, one phase possessing a low surface viscosity under stress and the other being present in the form of an elastic network.

If a small sphere is gently drawn off a cell membrane the remainder seals itself (Rand et al., 1964b), but Kochen (1965) has shown that in sudden haemolysis a rupture of the membrane can occur through which the haemoglobin escapes and has proposed a two-layer structure, the inner being predominantly elastic in behaviour and the outer mainly viscous (Kochen, 1967). This structure is reminiscent of the type suggested by Dintenfass (1964a) and mentioned above.

Cell Interior. About 32 per cent of the human red cell consists of haemoglobin (Pennell, 1964) and the form in which it is present is obviously very important in determining the physical properties of the cell. Polymeric solutions of mol. wt. 64,000 (the approximate value for haemoglobin) have a very high viscosity whereas Dintenfass (1962) deduced from a rheological analysis of blood behaviour that the internal viscosity was between 2 and 20 centipoise. It is possible that the haemoglobin is not in true solution but is suspended in a second phase or exists in an quasicrystalline form (Ponder, 1948; Bateman et al., 1953; Lehmann et al., 1961; Dintenfass, 1965a). From the ability of a red cell to regain its original shape after haemolysis it can be assumed that haemoglobin does not contribute structural strength to the shape of the red cell.

The Whole Cell. The red cell behaves as a polyanion when in suspension (Seaman et al., 1964) but this property can be removed or reversed by treatment with suitable reagents (Castaneda et al., 1964; Seaman et al., 1965a). Two physical properties of the cell which are particularly remarkable are its extreme flexibility and the bidiscoidal shape. They are related to some extent in that a change in shape or volume of any body is normally accompanied by an alteration in the rigidity. Such changes would lead to appreciable alterations in the area of the membrane if the cells were spherical but the bidiscoidal shape permits the membrane to deform and maintain a constant surface area. Rand et al. (1964b) found that the pressure difference across the membrane altered insignificantly as the cell transformed to a sphere during haemolysis and that the pressure inside a human cell was some 2·3 mm of water greater than outside. Such a pressure difference makes it difficult to understand how the concavities on the cell surface are able to maintain themselves. Assuming that the contours of the membrane determine the form of the cell it does not seem possible to make an elastic model which emulates the observed changes in shape with pressure (Burton, 1964). On the other hand, it does not appear to be controlled by the contents of the cell and the reason for its unique shape is still unresolved.

The remarkable flexibility of the cell is seen in the many photographs which have been taken of the microcirculation (Krogh, 1959; Bloch, 1962; Guest et al., 1963; Monro, 1964; Brånemark, 1965; Maggio, 1965). They can move easily through very narrow living capillaries (down to 3 μ in diameter) and through the pores of microfilters some 5 μ in size (Prothero et al., 1962b; Gregerson et al., 1967) but it is much more difficult to force them down glass tubes of less than 20 μ in diameter because of a strong adsorption of cell and plasma elements on the glass (Merrill et al., 1961) and the probable release of toxic substances (Strumia, 1964). On the other hand,

Burton (1965) has reported flow through glass orifices as small as 3 μ in diameter, the red cells curling or folding along a diameter. According to Teitel (1965), however, the ability of red cells to pass through small apertures depends not on their biconcave shape but on the ability of the membrane to undergo distortion. Thus the sphering of normal cells may have an insignificant effect on the size of aperture through which they can pass but in many cases a complex combination of flexing, distortion and elongation is undoubtedly involved (Brånemark, 1965).

White Cells. White cells, or leucocytes, are responsible for protecting the body from disease (Britton, 1963). They can be divided into three sizes varying from 16 to 22 μ for monocytes, to 10 to 12 μ for lymphocytes and granulocytes, although by a process of maturation the size of lymphocytes decreases to about 7 μ (Bell *et al.*, 1961). Under conditions of normal health their volume concentration in the blood is totally insignificant compared to the red cells, there being about one white to every 1000 red cells. Even in acute infection the increased number does not constitute a significant change. However, in cases of infection white cells may attach to vessel walls, reducing the effective cross-section area of flow (Macfarlane, 1961; Merrill *et al.*, 1961; Berman, 1964; Sanders *et al.*, 1966; Stehbens, 1967b) and seriously altering the flow pattern.

A white cell possesses a distensible, gelatinous membrane that can shrink and swell and may assume the shape which local conditions require. They seem to be more rigid than red cells because they have been observed to indent red cells on collision (Palmer, 1959; Brånemark *et al.*, 1963). This, it has been suggested, is because the material inside a white cell is more viscous and shear-dependent than the haemoglobin in a red cell (Dintenfass, 1965a).

Platelets. These are much smaller than red or white cells, being 2–3 μ in diameter (Bell *et al.*, 1961; Britton, 1963) although a value of only 0·5 μ has been quoted (Merrill *et al.*, 1961). The classic concept of a small platelike disc (Tuttle *et al.*, 1965), has been modified to include a membrane (Rhodin, 1967b; Stewart, 1967) and the important changes which occur in abnormal physiological environments include the projection of many small fibrils from the surface (Tullis, 1953; Macfarlane, 1961) and the development of granules in their structure (Stewart, 1967). Because the number of platelets present is only one-tenth of the red cells and each has a much smaller volume than a red cell, their direct effect on the resistance to flow of blood is probably insignificant. Indeed their volume concentration in normal blood has been given as only about 0·3 per cent (Britton, 1963). When they are damaged or are shed extravascularly or adsorb on broken tissue or on foreign surfaces, however, they liberate reagents which play important roles in the clotting reactions of the blood and profoundly alter its flow properties.

Plasma

Human blood plasma, the continuous liquid medium in which the particulate substances are suspended, consists of a solution of plasma proteins in an aqueous medium whose average analysis is shown in Table 2.5. Important anions other than chloride are also present

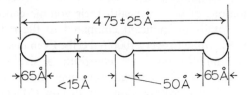

FIG. 2.7. Model of the fibrinogen molecule (after Hall *et al.*, 1959).

in small quantities, notably the buffering anions of citrate, bicarbonate, phosphate and sulphate (Merrill *et al.*, 1961). Proteins, constituting in total some 7 per cent of the total volume of the plasma, are found in this medium but although a bewildering number has been isolated they can be divided into three main groups according to the classical view (Bell *et al.*, 1961). These are:

FIBRINOGEN. This has one of the largest molecules of the plasma proteins and is the most asymmetric (see Table 2.6 and Fig. 2.7). The large asymmetry gives it an intrinsic viscosity of about 27 (Tanford, 1965) so that although it is present in relatively low concentration it makes a substantial contribution to the total viscosity of plasma (see Table 1.1). When blood clots in the absence of an anticoagulating agent the fibrinogen polymerizes to fibrin which contracts if the clot of fibrin and blood cells is left for some time. The fluid left behind contains the globulin and albumin protein factions and is termed the *serum*.

GLOBULINS. These have been divided into α, β and γ groups each of which contains sub-groups. The molecules cover a very wide

TABLE 2.5

Concentration of electrolytes in human plasma[1]

Cations	Plasma (m-equiv./l.)	Anions	Plasma (m-equiv./l.)
Na^+	145	Cl^-	103
K^{++}	4·2	HCO_3^-	29
Ca^{++}	4·8	Others	23·6
Mg^{++}	1·6		
	155·6		155·6

[1] Davson et al. (1962).

TABLE 2.6

Plasma proteins

Protein	Molecular weight	Shape	Dimensions (Å)	Concentration (g/100 ml)
Fibrinogen	340,000[1]	Dumbell†	475 × 50[2]	0·2–0·4[3, 4]
α Globulin	—	—	—	0·7–1·1[3, 4]
β Globulin	—	—	—	0·8–1·3[3, 4]
γ Globulin	160,000[5]	Ellipsoid	235 × 45[5]	0·6–0·9[3, 4]
Albumin	65–70,000[6]	Prism	150 × 50[5]	3·5–5·3[3, 4]

[1] Caspary and Kekwick. Quoted by Macfarlane (1960).
[2] Hall et al. (1959).
[3] Bell et al. (1961).
[4] Haurowitz (1961).
[5] Phelps et al. (1960).
[6] Foster (1960).
† See Fig. 2.7.

range of molecular weights—mostly from 40,000 to about one million according to Phelps et al. (1960)—and the specific functions of each are by no means completely understood. Their behaviour as carriers of lipids and other water-insoluble substances is extremely important (Haurowitz, 1961) and it is known that γ globulin contains the antibodies which resist infections from bacteria and viruses. The relative proportions of the various groups in normal health are shown in Table 2.6. Although they are present in greater concentrations than fibrinogen, the asymmetry (and thus the intrinsic viscosities) of the globulin molecules are usually much less.

ALBUMIN. This is the most abundant plasma protein and possesses the lowest molecular weight (Table 2.6). Because of these characteristics it is responsible for about 80 per cent of the total osmotic pressure of the plasma proteins and thus may be important in the balance of water metabolism, although this could have been overestimated (Haurowitz, 1961).

The sizes of the protein molecules are such that they are normally unable to pass through the capillary walls; in abnormal conditions the walls may become permeable to molecules of the size of albumin which probably escape through pores between the endothelial cells (Maggio, 1965). The low asymmetry of the molecule gives it a comparatively low intrinsic viscosity (see Table 1.1).

Plasma also contains widely varying amounts of emulsified fats, chloresterol, free fatty acids, adrenalin, dissolved oxygen and dissolved carbon dioxide, the concentrations of all of which alter with the conditions of the living system. Almost all the oxygen which is carried in the blood stream is within the red cell however, the oxygen-carrying capacity of plasma being only about $2\frac{1}{2}$ per cent of that of whole blood (Merrill et al., 1961).

CHAPTER 3

THE FLOW OF FLUIDS†

Types of Flow

In Chapter 1 the behaviour was examined of various materials when confined between flat parallel planes under the influence of a tangential stress. No internal restraining stresses are developed in the case of a fluid and the viscous drag, through which the energy supplied to the fluid is dissipated, is the result of the slippage of parallel layers of fluid over each other. The whole space between the planes can be imagined as filled with thin laminae of fluid (Fig. 3.1), resting on each other and moving at a velocity which is

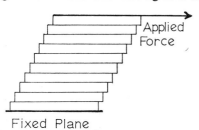

Applied Force

Fixed Plane

FIG. 3.1. Laminar (or viscous) flow.

proportional to their distance from the fixed plane. This type of flow is frequently called *laminar* or *viscous*.

In the more general case of the steady flow of a fluid at low velocity in the vicinity of a stationary solid surface it is possible to imagine continuous lines drawn through the fluid, tangents to which are at every point in the direction of flow (Fig. 3.2). Such lines are termed streamlines and the flow is called *streamline*: the energy of the fluid is still dissipated in viscous drag between adjacent laminae.

† Standard texts which cover parts of this subject include Goldstein (1938), Rouse (1946), Prandtl (1952), Pai (1956), Wilkinson (1960), Levich (1962), Daugherty *et al.* (1965).

If the velocity of the fluid is increased a value may be reached at which continuous streamlines cannot be followed by the fluid elements. They are not then retained in laminae but move in a heterogeneous fashion, sliding past some elements and colliding with others in an entirely haphazard manner, causing mixture of the fluid as flow occurs. During the mixing some elements of fluid are accelerated and others decelerated leading to direct transformation of some energy in the fluid to heat. These forces, which lead to a direct conversion of velocity energy to heat energy, are termed

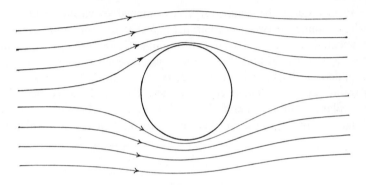

FIG. 3.2. Streamline flow round a cylinder.

inertial and should be distinguished from viscous forces by which velocity energy is translated to heat through the viscous drag between adjacent elements of fluid.

Turbulence can develop in any fluid if it undergoes a sudden change in direction or velocity of flow and it is most important to be able to specify the conditions under which turbulence may die out downstream of the disturbance and permit streamline flow to re-establish itself. This depends not only upon the geometry of the surrounding or interfering surfaces but also on the viscosity and density of the fluid. Moreover, the onset of turbulence is influenced by whether the flow is at a constant velocity or not. Reynolds realized that for a steady velocity the borderline between laminar and turbulent flow might be expressed numerically. He suggested that this borderline could be defined by a dimensionless combination of the velocity v, the viscosity η and the density ρ of the fluid, together with some characteristic dimension d_c of the flow region. The combination has become known as Reynolds number Re and takes the form

$$Re = \frac{v\, d_c\, \rho}{\eta}.$$

Two situations which have been carefully and extensively examined experimentally and are of particular interest in the case of blood, relate to flow in tubes and round certain obstacles. For a simple fluid in a cylindrical tube, v is normally taken as the mean velocity of flow $\bar{v}_t$ and d_c as the internal diameter of the tube d_i although the radius is occasionally used. Systematic experiments on Newtonian fluids by many observers have confirmed Reynolds' conclusions that if all disturbing sources such as roughness, vibration and sharp corners are eliminated at the entrance to the pipe, tube Reynolds numbers (Re_t) as high as 50,000 can be reached without the development of turbulence. In smooth pipes at tube Reynolds numbers exceeding about 2300 a certain disturbance is necessary to initiate stable turbulence and the larger the tube Reynolds number the smaller need the initial disturbance be. Below the critical value of 2300 any disturbance introduced into the flow may still cause local turbulence but this will be damped out as the fluid travels down the tube and laminar flow will ultimately be restored. The question of whether and under what conditions the flow of blood in living systems or *in vitro* is laminar or turbulent is one which has been examined very carefully by many haemodynamicists and will be discussed in detail in Chapter 7.

In the case of an immersed sphere or a circular plate held normal to the flow, the characteristic dimension d_c is generally taken as the diameter. With this dimension the Reynolds number required for the initiation of a turbulent wake is approximately $0 \cdot 5$ for Newtonian fluids but its appearance is not so well defined as the onset of stable turbulence in a tube. Measurable deviations in flow resistance from streamline conditions begin at a Reynolds number of about $0 \cdot 5$ and are appreciable by the time a value of 1 or 2 is reached.

Flow in Tubes

Newtonian Fluids

Laminar Flow. Consider a rigid, straight, cylindrical tube of radius R_i down which a Newtonian fluid is flowing with constant velocity (Fig. 3.3). It is assumed that entrance effects can be ignored and that the fluid is at rest in contact with the tube wall. In order to maintain the flow there must be a pressure gradient down the tube but because there is no radial flow the pressure will be constant

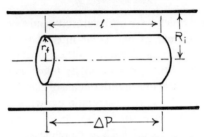

FIG. 3.3. Fluid flowing in a cylindrical tube.

across any section of the tube. Let the pressure difference be ΔP over a length l of the tube. The pressure gradient $= \Delta P/l$. Consider a cylinder of the fluid of unit length and radius r_f situated on the tube axis. The difference in force between the ends of the cylinder $= (\Delta P/l)\,\pi r_f^2$. The opposing force comes from the viscous drag on the surface of the cylinder. If the tangential stress $= \tau$,

$$\text{Viscous drag force} = \tau\,.\,2\pi r_f\,.\,1.$$

For the velocity to be steady,

$$\frac{\Delta P}{l}\,.\,\pi r_f^2 = \tau\,.\,2\pi r_f$$

or, $$\tau = \frac{\Delta P r_f}{2l}. \tag{3.1}$$

At the tube wall $r_f = R_i$ and the shear stress τ_w is given by

$$\tau_w = \frac{\Delta P R_i}{2l}. \tag{3.2}$$

Now the coefficient of viscosity of the fluid η is defined by

$$\eta = \frac{\tau}{D}. \tag{1.3}$$

The rate of shear D changes continuously with tube radius from zero on the axis to a maximum at the wall. It equals the velocity gradient dv_N/dr_f at radius r_f because the lines of shear are not curved.

Since v_N decreases as r_f increases

$$D = -\frac{dv_N}{dr_f}$$

and

$$\tau = -\eta \frac{dv_N}{dr_f}. \qquad (3.3)$$

Substituting eqn. (3.3) in eqn. (3.1) and simplifying,

$$dv_N = -\frac{\Delta P}{2l\eta} \cdot r_f \, dr_f.$$

Integrating and using the boundary conditions that $v_N = 0$ when $r_f = R_i$

$$v_N = \frac{\Delta P}{4l\eta}(R_i^2 - r_f^2). \qquad (3.4)$$

Thus the velocity profile is parabolic as shown in Fig. 3.4.

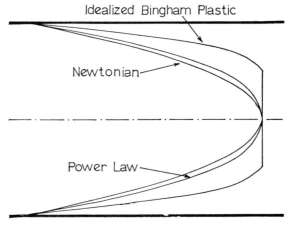

FIG. 3.4. Velocity profiles of different materials in streamline flow in a cylindrical tube.

Now consider a cylindrical annulus of fluid of inner radius r_f and thickness dr_f (Fig. 3.5).

The quantity of fluid flowing down the annulus in unit time q is given by

$$q = v_N \cdot 2\pi r_f \, dr_f.$$

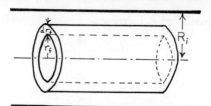

FIG. 3.5. A fluid annulus in a cylindrical tube.

Substituting for v_N from eqn. (3.4) and integrating from $r_f = 0$ to $r_f = R_i$, the total flow rate is given by

$$Q_N = \frac{\Delta P \pi R_i{}^4}{8l\eta}. \tag{3.5}$$

This is known as the *Poiseuille* equation.

If the mean velocity of flow in the tube $= \bar{v}_t$

$$Q_N = \pi R_i{}^2 . \bar{v}_t$$

so that
$$\bar{v}_t = \frac{\Delta P R_i{}^2}{8l\eta}. \tag{3.6}$$

The rate of shear at the wall D_w is found from eqn. (1.3)

$$D_w = \frac{\tau_w}{\eta}.$$

Substituting for τ_w from eqn. (3.2)

$$D_w = \frac{\Delta P R_i}{2l\eta}. \tag{3.7}$$

The mean rate of shear across the tube D_t is given by

$$\bar{D}_t = \frac{\displaystyle\int_0^{R_i} D . 2\pi r_f \, dr_f}{\pi R_i{}^2}.$$

Substituting for D from eqn. (1.3) and using eqn. (3.1)

$$\bar{D}_t = \frac{\Delta P R_i}{3l\eta} = \frac{2}{3} D_w. \tag{3.8}$$

Equations (3.2)–(3.8) inclusive are useful for calculating various parameters of viscous flow in tubes.

Turbulent Flow. Because turbulence represents chaotic motion of small fluid elements through short distances in every direction when flow takes place, the motion of individual elements is impossible to characterize mathematically. But mathematical relationships may be obtained by considering the average motion of aggregates of fluid elements or by statistical methods.

The velocity distribution in a circular pipe is no longer parabolic as in laminar flow (Fig. 3.4) but much more nearly uniform near the centre of the pipe, with a very steep gradient near the walls. As the tube Reynolds number increases, the velocity distribution over the cross-section becomes more and more uniform. The average velocity $\bar{v}_t$ is no longer proportional to the pressure gradient $\Delta P/l$ as in eqn. (3.6) but increases at a slower rate.

The calculation of pressure gradient in a tube under turbulent flow is more difficult than when the flow is laminar and requires the application of various approximations. Fortunately full turbulence probably occurs in only a few of the largest blood vessels and a full discussion of the calculation problems is inappropriate here. If the tube walls can be considered smooth the most satisfactory method is as follows:

(1) Calculate the tube Reynolds number of the flow, assuming

$$Re_t = \frac{\bar{v}_t\, d_i\, \rho}{\eta}.$$

(2) Use the Blasius equation $f = \dfrac{0 \cdot 3164}{Re_t^{\frac{1}{4}}}$ to obtain an approximate value of the *friction coefficient f*. This is a dimensionless group which includes the pressure gradient $\Delta P/l$ as one of its terms [see eqn. (3.10) below].

(3) Substitute the approximate value of f in the right-hand side of the *universal pipe-law* equation

$$\frac{1}{\sqrt{f}} = 2 \log_{10} (Re \sqrt{f}) - 0 \cdot 8. \tag{3.9}$$

This results in a new value of f which can be resubstituted in the right-hand side of eqn. (3.9) to give a second value for f. Normally a single repetition will give a sufficiently accurate value.

(4) Calculate the pressure gradient from

$$\frac{\Delta P}{l} = \frac{f \, \bar{v}_t^2}{4 \, R_i}. \tag{3.10}$$

The reader should refer to one of the many standard textbooks on fluid mechanics for alternative methods of calculating flow in tubes under conditions of turbulence.

Non-Newtonian Fluids

Fluids which do not exhibit a constant relationship between shear stress and rate of shear can follow a variety of other flow equations. Those most generally applicable to the case of blood assume that it behaves either as a power-law fluid (p. 7) or a Bingham plastic (p. 9). It should be noted, however, that although blood differs in its flow properties from a Newtonian fluid, the divergence is not great compared with that of many practical liquids and suspensions.

If the flow of a non-Newtonian fluid down a straight cylindrical tube is laminar, a similar derivation to that used for Newtonian fluids leads to equations for the velocity profile and the flow rate.

Power-Law Fluid. It was mentioned on page 7 that this follows the equation

$$K_{pl} = \frac{\tau}{D^s} \tag{1.4}$$

where s is a constant and K_{pl} is a measure of the consistency of the fluid.

For the velocity of flow v_{pl} at radius r_f from the tube axis, the Newtonian equation (3.4) is replaced by

$$v_{pl} = \left(\frac{s}{s+1}\right) \left(\frac{\Delta P}{2lK_{pl}}\right)^{1/s} \left(R_i^{(s+1)/s} - r_f^{(s+1)/s}\right). \tag{3.11}$$

It will be observed that the velocity profile is not parabolic, but depends upon the value of s. For suspensions of red cells s is approximately equal to $0 \cdot 75$ (p. 73) and the velocity profile, from eqn. (3.11) is as shown in Fig. 3.4. By differentiating eqn. (3.11) the rate of shear is obtained and it can easily be shown that the mean rate of shear across the tube for a suspension of red cells is then $0 \cdot 60$ of the shear rate at the wall, compared with $0 \cdot 67$ if the suspension were Newtonian and obeyed eqn. (3.8).

The flow rate down the tube

$$Q_{pl} = \frac{s\pi R_i^3}{3s+1}\left(\frac{\Delta P R_i}{2lK_{pl}}\right)^{1/s}$$ (3.12)

and replaces eqn. (3.5) which is applicable to a Newtonian fluid.

Various parameters have been suggested for the onset of turbulence but as yet no completely reliable criterion has emerged. Most of them rely on a modified tube Reynolds number which includes the two rheological parameters of the liquid, K_{pl} and s (Wilkinson, 1960; Bogue et al., 1963).

Bingham Plastic. This follows the equation

$$\eta_p = \frac{\tau - \tau_y}{D}$$ (1.7)

where η_p and τ_y are the plastic viscosity and the yield stress respectively. In this case the velocity at distance r from the tube axis is given by

$$v_B = \frac{1}{\eta_p}\left[\frac{\Delta P(R_i^2 - r_f^2)}{4l} - \tau_y(R_i - r_f)\right].$$ (3.13)

The velocity profile is then as shown in Fig. 3.4, the diameter of the central unsheared plug decreasing with increasing velocity of flow and becoming almost parabolic at high flow rates. If $\Delta P/l < 2\tau_y/R_i$ the plug fills the whole cross-section and no flow is possible but if it is exceeded the flow rate down the tube,

$$Q_B = \frac{\Delta P\pi R_i^4}{8l\eta_p}\left[1 - \frac{4}{3}\left(\frac{2l\tau_y}{\Delta P R_i}\right) + \frac{1}{3}\left(\frac{2l\tau_y}{\Delta P R_i}\right)^4\right].$$ (3.14)

This is known as Buckingham's equation and it replaces Poiseuille's equation (3.5) for an idealized Bingham plastic.

It has already been mentioned that very few (if indeed any) materials possess the properties of an idealized Bingham plastic and blood is not unusual in this respect. Consequently considerable errors can be introduced by using eqns. (3.13) and (3.14) particularly at low rates of shear and a better fit is given for whole blood by using the empirical Casson equation

$$K_C = \frac{\sqrt{\tau} - \sqrt{\tau_y}}{\sqrt{D}}$$ (1.8)

where K_C is a measure of the consistency of the fluid. It has been shown on a number of occasions (Reiner *et al.*, 1959; Oka, 1965; Merrill *et al.*, 1965a) that eqn. (3.4) for the velocity of the fluid at distance r_f from the tube axis is replaced by

$$v_C = \frac{\Delta P}{4lK_C{}^2}\left(R_i{}^2 - r_f{}^2\right) - \frac{4\sqrt{\tau_y}}{3\ K_C{}^2}\left(\frac{\Delta P}{2l}\right)^{1/2}\left(R_i{}^{3/2} - r_f{}^{3/2}\right)$$

$$+ \frac{\tau_y}{K_C{}^2}\left(R_i - r_f\right). \tag{3.15}$$

The velocity profile is similar in form to that for an idealized Bingham plastic but different in detail. The flow rate down the tube is given by

$$Q_C = \frac{\Delta P \pi R_i{}^4}{8lK_C{}^2}\left[1 - \frac{16}{7}\left(\frac{2l\tau_y}{\Delta P R_i}\right)^{1/2} + \frac{4}{3}\left(\frac{2l\tau_y}{\Delta P R_i}\right)\right.$$

$$\left. - \frac{1}{21}\left(\frac{2l\tau_y}{\Delta P R_i}\right)^4\right]. \tag{3.16}$$

This equation is only valid if $\Delta P/l > 2\tau_y/R_i$, as in the case of an idealized Bingham plastic.

It should be noted that eqns. (3.14) and (3.16) cannot be solved explicitly for the pressure gradient $\Delta P/l$ if the flow rate is known and that both reduce to the Poiseuille equation when $\tau_y = 0$.

The onset of turbulence in Bingham plastics is difficult to define but it has been determined from a modified Reynolds number in which the viscosity of a simple liquid was replaced by the plastic viscosity of the Bingham plastic (Valentik *et al.*, 1965). The contribution of the yield stress to the flow resistance is small when the flow becomes fully turbulent but the Reynolds number at which stable turbulence develops tends to increase as the yield stress increases.

CHAPTER 4

VISCOMETRY†

In Chapter 1 the properties of fluids were described on the assumption that they could be held between parallel planes of infinite extent and that geometrically simple shearing forces could be applied to precise volumes of them by tangential movement of the planes relative to one another. These assumptions ignore the problems of edge effects to which the material would be exposed if practical measurements were attempted in this way and of maintaining continuous shear in a preselected volume of fluid.

Very many instruments have been designed which overcome these difficulties and some of them are suitable for measuring the flow properties of blood and plasma. They can in general be reduced to two broad categories—rotational and tube instruments. A third category, in which the resistance of the fluid to a body moving through it is measured, has also appeared in various forms of falling-sphere and Pocchetino viscometers (Copley *et al.*, 1942; Burgman *et al.*, 1964) but these instruments have been limited in their use by the difficulty of specifying precisely the rate of shear to which the fluid is exposed. Also measurements of the resistance to flow of blood through a fine screen have been made (Swank *et al.*, 1964) but the information obtained relates primarily to the degree or form of aggregation in the blood rather than to its viscosity.

There follows a brief description of the operating principles and characteristics of the main categories of viscometer. Detailed information on the various types of instruments is readily available elsewhere (Barr, 1931; Merrington, 1949; Oka, 1960; Reiner 1960; Dinsdale *et al.*, 1962; Van Wazer *et al.*, 1963).

Rotational Viscometers

Essentially these consist of two members, separated by the material under test, which rotate relative to one another about a common

† Standard texts dealing with viscometry include Barr (1931), Merrington (1949), Dinsdale *et al.* (1962) and Van Wazer *et al.* (1963).

vertical axis. The rotation of one member tends to drag the other round with it, the relationship between the angular velocity of the rotating member and the torque developed on the other characterizing the viscous properties of the fluid. The two main types are the co-axial cylinder and the cone plate.

Co-axial Cylinder Type

The fluid is held in a cylindrical pot containing a concentrically mounted bob (Fig. 4.1). The pot is rotated at a constant velocity

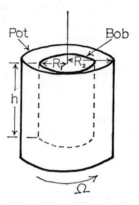

FIG. 4.1. Co-axial rotating cylinder viscometer.

and the viscous drag transmitted through the fluid is measured by the angular deflection of the inner cylinder (if it is suspended from a wire) or by the force required to return it to its original position. This arrangement was originally used by Couette after whom it is named. Occasionally the bob is rotated and the drag transmitted to the pot is recorded but in both cases the geometry approximates to the ideal of two flat planes moving parallel to one another and the approximation improves as the radii of the cylinders are increased and the width of the intervening annulus is reduced.

Corrections have to be made for drag transmitted between the base of the bob and the base of the pot, and sometimes for the presence of a free surface to the fluid under test which may lead to the transmission of surface forces brought about by, for example the denaturing of plasma (Merrill *et al.*, 1963a). Whitmore (1960a) showed that if the fluid consisted of a suspension of dispersed particles in a liquid any redistribution of the particles across the annulus should not alter the transmitted torque, provided that the flow approximated closely to that between flat parallel planes and the suspension obeyed the equation (Oliver *et al.*, 1953)

$$\eta_r = \frac{1}{1 - K_1 c}. \tag{4.1}$$

Unfortunately although eqn. (4.1) satisfies many suspensions up to a concentration of about 30 per cent, it will be shown in Chapter 6 that blood is probably an exception so that a radial movement of red cells away from the viscometer walls could influence the measured viscosity. Sometimes grooved cylinders are used in order to ensure that the fluid cannot slip at the surface and this is particularly necessary if the material possesses an appreciable yield stress.

Newtonian Fluid. For a Newtonian fluid shearing under laminar flow conditions the torque transmitted to the inner cylinder is given by

$$T = \frac{4 \pi R_1^2 R_2^2 h \eta \Omega}{R_2^2 - R_1^2} \tag{4.2}$$

where R_1 = radius of inner cylinder, R_2 = radius of outer cylinder, h = height of inner cylinder, and Ω = angular velocity of outer cylinder.

Thus for a given viscometer geometry and at a constant angular velocity the torque transmitted is proportional to the viscosity of the fluid. This is the basis of the calibration method of using a rotating cylinder viscometer. The torques transmitted by fluids of known viscosity at a constant angular velocity are measured and a calibration curve constructed. The viscosity of an unknown fluid can then be found from the torque which it transmits at a predetermined angular velocity.

The arithmetic mean shear stress $\bar{\tau}$ is given by

$$\bar{\tau} = T \left(\frac{R_1^2 + R_2^2}{4 \pi h R_1^2 R_2^2} \right) \tag{4.3}$$

and the corresponding mean shear rate $\bar{D}$ by

$$\bar{D} = \Omega \left(\frac{R_1^2 + R_2^2}{R_2^2 - R_1^2} \right). \tag{4.4}$$

It should be noted that eqns. (4.3) and (4.4) are equally applicable when the inner cylinder is rotated and the outer cylinder is at rest.

For non-Newtonian fluids the shearing stress τ is no longer directly proportional to the rate of shear D as required by eqn. (1.3) and thus the measured torque T is not directly proportional to the angular velocity Ω. Equations (4.2), (4.3), and (4.4) become inapplicable and others take their place.

Power-Law Fluid. For a power-law fluid [eqn. (1.4)] the transmitted torque is given by

$$T = 2 \pi h R_1^2 R_2^2 \left[\frac{2 \Omega K_{pl}}{s (R_2^{2/s} - R_1^{2/s})} \right]^s . \tag{4.5}$$

Equation (4.5) reduces to eqn. (4.1) when $s = 1$ because the fluid is then Newtonian. The slope of a logarithmic plot of T against Ω gives the value of s, and the intercept at $\log_{10} T = 0$ leads directly to the value of K_{pl} if end effects are ignored. It is usually more simple, however, to calibrate the viscometer with Newtonian fluids and thus obtain a series of apparent viscosities η_a for the power-law fluid at different known rates of shear. The applied shear stress τ at each rate of shear D can then be obtained from the equation

$$D = \frac{\tau}{\eta_a} . \tag{4.6}$$

A logarithmic plot of τ against D is made and s and K_{pl} obtained from eqn. (1.4).

Bingham Plastic. Three different shearing conditions may prevail in the viscometer annulus.

(a) If $T < 2\pi R_1^2 h \tau_y$, the shearing stress throughout the material in the viscometer is less than the yield stress and no shear occurs.

(b) If $2\pi R_1^2 h \tau_y < T < 2\pi R_2^2 h \tau_y$, the shearing stress exceeds the yield stress only in the region between the inner cylinder and a critical radius R_c. Thus shear occurs in the material between the inner cylinder and R_c while the material between R_c and the outer cylinder behaves as a solid shell as shown in Fig. 4.2. R_c increases with the angular velocity of the cylinders.

(c) If $T > 2\pi R_2^2 h \tau_y$, the shearing stress exceeds the yield stress at all points and all the material between the cylinders is sheared.

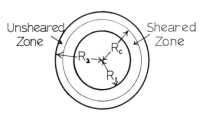

FIG. 4.2. Bingham plastic under shear in a co-axial rotating cylinder
viscometer.

In a well-designed viscometer the range of torque corresponding to
the intermediate region of flow (b) should be only a small fraction
of the total range.

In the flow region (c) a plot of τ against D is linear for an idealized
Bingham plastic [eqn. (1.7)] while if the Casson equation is followed
[eqn. (1.8)] $\sqrt{\tau}$ increases linearly with $\sqrt{D}$. The plastic viscosity
η_p and consistency constant K_C respectively are obtained from the
slopes of the two curves while the yield stress is found from the
extrapolation of the linear portions of the respective curves to $D = 0$.

Unspecified Fluids. If the relationship between τ and D is initially
unknown the usual method is to calculate the arithmetic mean shearing stress $\bar{\tau}$ for each experimental point from eqn. (4.3), together
with the quantity y where

$$y = \frac{\Omega}{\bar{\tau}}.$$

The true shear rate is then given by Mooney's equation (Dinsdale
et al., 1962)

$$D = \frac{\bar{D}}{K_3} - \frac{\bar{\tau}^3 K_3 d^2 y}{(6 + 2K_3^2)d\bar{\tau}^2} + \frac{\bar{\tau}^4 K_3^3}{(9 + 12K_3^2 + 3K_3^4)} \cdot \frac{d^3 y}{d\bar{\tau}^3} \qquad (4.7)$$

where $K_3 = (R_2^2 - R_1^2)/(R_1^2 + R_2^2)$.

The second and third terms are correction terms, the second being
obtained by repeated graphical or numerical differentiation; the
third term is rarely required.

Cone-plate Type

The fluid is contained in the space between a cone of very large
apex angle and a flat surface normal to its axis (Fig. 4.3). One unit

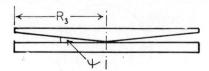

FIG. 4.3. Cone-plate viscometer.

is rotated and the drag transmitted by the fluid is measured on the other. It is apparent from the geometry of the system that the perpendicular distance between the cone and the plate increases proportionally with the radius. Moreover the linear relative velocity of the cone or the plate also increases proportionally with radius so that the rate of shear in the fluid is constant throughout. Because the cone angle is very large (usually at least 178°) the volume of fluid required is small but it is uncertain whether the presence of a free surface of fluid can, in some cases, affect the transmitted torque.

If ψ = angle between cone and plate (in radians) and R_3 = radius of the cone and the plate

$$\text{The rate of shear } D = \frac{\Omega}{\psi} . \qquad (4.8)$$

$$\text{The shear stress } \tau = \frac{3T}{2\pi R_3^2} . \qquad (4.9)$$

Thus, for a Newtonian fluid

$$\eta = \frac{3T \, \psi}{2\pi R_3^2 \Omega} .$$

Equations (4.8) and (4.9) are generally used without correction for plotting flow curves of non-Newtonian fluids (Dinsdale *et al.*, 1962), the viscometer first being calibrated with Newtonian fluids of known viscosity. The apparent viscosity of the unknown non-Newtonian fluid is then found at various rates of shear and the corresponding shear stress obtained from eqn. (4.6). The flow curve can then be constructed immediately.

There have been reports of circulation developing between the cone and the plate during the shearing of certain non-Newtonian fluids and suspensions, leading to incorrect results (Hoppmann *et al.*, 1964; Highgate, 1966). In the case of a dispersed suspension which obeys eqn. (4.1), any redistribution of the particles perpendicular to the direction of shear should not affect the measurement of the viscosity of the suspension (Charm *et al*., 1962) but aggregated suspensions often behave as Bingham plastics, in which case complications can occur in the shearing pattern at low rates of shear and it may be difficult to calculate the true parameters of the material, particularly the yield stress (Boardman *et al*., 1963).

Tube Viscometers†

The fluid is allowed to flow from a reservoir down a tube of precisely known dimensions and the volume conveyed in a given time under a given pressure difference is recorded. Precision-bore glass or steel tubing is generally used and, in the case of blood, it is often less than 100 μ in diameter in order for the flow to be streamline and the pressure difference reasonably large. If the tube is too narrow, however, the recorded viscosity of heterogeneous suspensions such as blood may become dependent upon the diameter of the tube; this phenomenon is discussed in Chapter 8. Corrections may be required for flow pattern changes and anomalous pressure gradients at the inlet and outlet to the tube while meniscus effects may also be present in some instruments (Jacobs, 1966). Although the rate of shear is not bounded by narrow limits as in a rotational instrument but varies from a maximum at the tube wall to zero on the axis, the flow curve of a homogeneous non-Newtonian fluid can still be established from data relating the flow rate down the tube to the ruling pressure gradient.

Newtonian Fluid. The viscosity of a Newtonian fluid can be obtained from Poiseuille's equation (see p. 42)

$$\eta = \frac{\Delta P \pi R^4{}_i}{8 l Q_N}.\tag{3.5}$$

It requires the tube radius R_i to be known with considerable precision, and corrections may be required for end effects at the inlet and outlet of the tube. These problems are largely avoided if the viscometer is calibrated by measuring the volume flow rate of New-tonian fluids of known viscosity and density under given pressure differences. The viscosity of an unknown fluid can then be found

† The alternative term "capillary-tube viscometer" is often used in the literature, particularly if the tube possesses a small bore and thick walls. In order to avoid confusion with the capillaries of living vessels the term "tube viscometer" is used in this book for instruments constructed from non-biological materials.

from its volume flow rate at the same pressure difference on the assumption that the end effects are unaltered.

Power-Law Fluid. The appropriate equation, which was given on page 45 is

$$Q_{pl} = \frac{s\pi R_i^3}{3s+1} \left(\frac{\Delta P R_i}{2l\,K_{pl}}\right)^{1/s}.$$ (3.12)

Taking logarithms,

$$\log_{10} Q_{pl} = \frac{1}{s}\log_{10}\frac{\Delta P}{l} + \log_{10}\left[\frac{s\pi R_i^{(3s+1)/s}}{(3s+1)(2K_{pl})^{1/s}}\right].$$

Thus a logarithmic plot of Q_{pl} against $\Delta P/l$ is a straight line whose slope,

$$\frac{\log_{10} Q_{pl}}{\log_{10}(\Delta P/l)} = \frac{1}{s}.$$

At $\log_{10} Q_{pl} = 0$, the intercept $= \log_{10}\left[\frac{s\pi R_i^{(3s+1)/s}}{(3s+1)(2K_{pl})^{1/s}}\right].$

On substituting the value of s already obtained, K_{pl} can be found immediately.

Bingham Plastic. If the material obeys the Casson equation the appropriate relationship, which was given on page 46 is

$$Q_c = \frac{\Delta P \pi R_i^4}{8l K_c^2}\left[1 - \frac{16}{7}\left(\frac{2l\tau_y}{\Delta P R_i}\right)^{1/2} + \frac{4}{3}\left(\frac{2l\tau_y}{\Delta P R_i}\right)\right.$$
$$\left. - \frac{1}{21}\left(\frac{2l\tau_y}{\Delta P R_i}\right)^4\right].$$ (3.16)

Equation (3.16) is difficult to use as it stands but Merrill *et al.* (1965a) showed that an approximation to it was very satisfactory for blood. Using this,

$$\left(\frac{\Delta P R_i}{2l}\right)^{1/2} = \tau_y^{1/2} + 2K_c\left(\frac{Q_c}{\pi R_i^3}\right)^{1/2}.$$ (4.10)

Thus a plot of $\sqrt{Q_c}$ against $\sqrt{(\Delta P/l)}$ should be a straight line from whose slope K_c can be obtained and whose intercept at $\Delta P/l = 0$ gives $\sqrt{\tau_y}$.

Unspecified Fluids. If there is no prior knowledge of the form of relationship between shear stress and the rate of shear, the best procedure is to plot $\tau_w = \Delta P R_i / 2l$ against $D_w = 4Q/\pi R_i^3$. As before, τ_w is the shearing stress at the wall of the tube and D_w would be the rate of shear at the wall if the material were Newtonian. Provided that the flow is streamlined and that there is no slippage at the wall the plot of τ_w against D_w is independent of the dimensions of the viscometer for a non-Newtonian liquid. The true relationship between τ and D can be found by correcting D_w according to the equation (Dinsdale et al., 1962)

$$D = \frac{3}{4} D_w + \frac{1}{4} \tau_w \frac{dD_w}{d\tau_w}.$$

Selection of Instrument

The tube viscometer has been used extensively for work on blood because it is cheap to buy or construct, requires only a small volume of fluid, is easy to use and gives good reproducibility. Moreover it simulates *extra vivum*, to some degree, the flow of blood *in vivo*. The primary disadvantages are that in the case of non-Newtonian fluids each viscosity measurement covers a wide range of shear rate for which allowance has to be made and, if the tube is too narrow, wall effects may influence the results obtained.

The co-axial cylinder viscometer has the advantage of shearing the great proportion of the fluid at something approaching a constant rate of shear. On the other hand, end effects on the cylinder are sometimes difficult to overcome or allow for, particularly in the case of non-Newtonian fluids. A well-designed instrument is expensive, particularly if it is to work on small samples of fluid at low rates of shear (which is often necessary in the case of blood).

The cone-plate viscometer possesses many of the advantages of the co-axial cylinder instrument and, in addition, normally requires a smaller sample. A disadvantage is that the distance over which shearing takes place may be so small that the discontinuous nature of a fluid such as blood could affect the magnitude of the transmitted stress. The long length and short width of the air–fluid interface at the perimeter of the shearing surfaces may also, in certain circumstances, affect stress transmission unless it can be allowed for by the inclusion of a guard ring or other special design features.

It should be particularly noted that even in well designed viscometers the ideal of shearing a fluid between flat parallel planes of infinite extent is only approximately satisfied and that various corrections must normally be applied to absolute viscometer readings. The main attraction of calibrating a viscometer with fluids of known viscosity is that it becomes possible to deduce the viscosity of an unknown fluid directly. The danger is that if the unknown fluid is Newtonian but possesses, for example, a different density or molecular structure from that of the test fluids, the correction terms may be altered and the fluid will be incorrectly classified as non-Newtonian. This problem is aggravated if the unknown fluid is, in fact, non-Newtonian because the relevant corrections may well be changed.

The general trend in the case of work on the intrinsic flow behaviour of blood is towards the wider application of rotating viscometers and away from tube instruments. For sophisticated rheological measurements of the elastico-viscous properties of blood and plasma, rotational instruments capable of oscillatory motion may be necessary although their use at present on biological systems is very limited and interpretation of the results presents difficulties if the cone-plate geometry is employed (Maude *et al.*, 1964; Nally, 1965). For routine and comparative work on blood and plasma the tube instrument is still widely employed and gives satisfactory results.

It is interesting to note that although most of the reported work using rotating viscometers has been made at shear rates of less than about 250 sec^{-1} the rate of shear in some of the vessels of many living mammals may be more than twice as great as this (see Chapter 7).

CHAPTER 5

RHEOLOGY OF PLASMA

BEFORE any direct physical measurements can be made on plasma it must usually be separated from the other constituents of the blood. This is achieved by sedimentation under the influence of gravitational or centrifugal force when the cellular material separates out in a lower layer with the plasma on top. However, as soon as blood is removed from a living body the normal clotting mechanism initiates the fibrinogen–fibrin transformation process and the rheology of the blood changes continuously until the clot is finally formed (see Chapter 6). It is usual, therefore to add an anticoagulating agent to the fresh blood, of which heparin,† sequestrene,‡ oxalate,§ or citrate‖ are the most popular. The anticoagulant should be isotonic and is sometimes prepared as an aqueous solution when

† *Heparin*: a polysaccharide (Britton, 1963) which is frequently used dry at a concentration of 0·1–0·2 mg/ml of blood (Dacie, 1956) but has been employed in the form of an aqueous solution at a concentration of 0·4 mg/ml of isotonic saline (Copley, 1960), when the blood was diluted by about 25 per cent. It is thought to neutralize thrombin in the presence of a co-factor located in the albumin fraction of serum (Dacie, 1956).

‡ *Sequestrene* (EDTA): consists of the disodium or dipotassium salt of ethylenediamine tetra-acetic acid, which is effective at a concentration of 1·0–2·0 mg/ml of blood (Darmady *et al.*, 1963). It is non-toxic and removes calcium which is essential to coagulation. Three per cent and 10 per cent aqueous solutions are generally employed giving a dilution of less than 4 per cent in the blood.

§ *Oxalate*: a mixed salt containing 60 per cent ammonium oxalate and 40 per cent potassium oxalate is usually used in a 2 per cent solution at a concentration of 2 mg/ml of blood (Darmady *et al.*, 1963). It precipitates the calcium as insoluble calcium oxalate (Britton, 1963) but is toxic and dilutes the blood by about 10 per cent.

‖ (i) *Citrate:* trisodium citrate in the form of an aqueous 4 per cent solution is effective at a concentration of 2·0–4·0 mg/ml of blood by binding the free calcium ions to the citrate radical (Britton, 1963). Unfortunately cell shrinkage is observed with this reagent and it has been largely abandoned.

(ii) *Acid-citrate-dextrose* (ACD): contains approximately equal proportions by weight of sodium citrate and glucose (Britton, 1963; Darmady *et al.*, 1963). It is used in a 5 per cent suspension at a concentration of 10–15 mg/ml of blood, the blood being diluted by about 25 per cent. This is the anticoagulant generally employed for the storage of blood.

the distilled water which is added with the agent dilutes the blood, alters the plasma viscosity and reduces the haematocrit.

Human plasma is a transparent, slightly yellowish fluid whose density is about 1·035 g/ml (Merrill *et al.*, 1961).

Viscosity

The viscosities of normal mammalian plasmas generally lie between 0·011 and 0·016 poise, falling with increasing temperature. The presence of the protein fractions (Table 2.6) is the major cause of the increased viscosity over the aqueous suspending medium (Table 2.5) and the diluting effects of most anticoagulants (which behave as simple liquids and possess lower viscosities than plasma) must therefore be taken into consideration. The general evidence is that they reduce the viscosity level but the magnitude of the change is by no means certain. Heparin apparently reduces the viscosity by up to 10 per cent (Copley, 1960; Merrill *et al.*, 1961; Cerny *et al.*, 1962; Charm *et al.*, 1962) but the actions of oxalate and citrate are conflicting. In some cases they reduce viscosity more than heparin (Merrill *et al.*, 1961; Gelin, 1965); in other cases the reduction is less (Copley, 1960) or absent (Charm *et al.*, 1962) but the results are blurred by uncertainty regarding the normal flow properties of plasma, the extent to which samples drawn from different animals are comparable and differences in experimental technique. Eckstein *et al.* (1941) and Mayer *et al.* (1965) concluded that blood viscosity (and presumably plasma viscosity also) was unchanged by the addition of dry heparin while sequestrene was reported to behave in a similar manner (Mayer *et al.*, 1965).

If it were known for certain that plasma possessed the properties of a Newtonian liquid a single viscosity figure would categorize its flow properties. However, there is no general agreement on its flow characteristics and anomalous behaviour has often been reported, generally as a rise in apparent viscosity with decreasing rate of shear.

Non-Newtonian Characteristics

Until a few years ago practically all viscosity measurements (with the notable exception of those by Brundage, 1934), were made in tube instruments and insufficient results were reported for the shear stress/rate of shear characteristics of plasma to be determined.

Most of the experimenters concluded that mammalian plasmas were non-Newtonian (Copley, 1960; Charm et al., 1962; Cerny, 1963) and recent measurements using rotating (Peric, 1963; Rand et al., 1964a; Gelin et al., 1965; Gregerson et al., 1965; Shorthouse et al., 1967) and Pocchetino (Burgman et al., 1964) viscometers have confirmed this. There is a distinct tendency for the non-Newtonian behaviour of plasma to increase as the general viscosity level rises and because the concentration of the proteins is a prime factor in determining the viscosity level it would seem to be responsible, partially or completely, for the observed non-Newtonian character-istics. From this argument it follows that some pathological plasmas should be highly non-Newtonian and a sample from a patient suffering from multiple myeloma and containing over four times the normal globulin content has been found to conform to this pattern (Thompson, 1964).

In contrast, other workers have found plasma to be Newtonian when measured in tube viscometers (Bingham et al., 1944; Merrill et al., 1965a) and this conclusion has also been supported by rotating viscometer work (Brundage, 1934; Merrill et al., 1963a; Chien et al., 1966). Seaman (1967) observed that the velocity of a red cell sus-pended in plasma in an electrophoresis cell was proportional to the potential difference across the electrodes, which again suggests New-tonian characteristics.

If the experimental evidence makes it impossible to conclude whether, and under what conditions, plasma is Newtonian theoreti-cal guidance is equally uncertain. The presence of highly asymmetric protein molecules like fibrinogen (Fig. 2.7) might lead to an incon-stant viscosity through a change in the mean orientation of the molecules with alterations in the rate of shear (p. 14). For low con-centrations of rigid molecules possessing the aspect ratio of fibrino-gen, Scheraga's calculations (1955) show that any fall in viscosity originating from increased orientation of the molecules is less than 2 per cent unless the rate of shear exceeds the rotary diffusion con-stant. Taking a value of about 38,000 for the rotary diffusion con-stant (Tanford, 1965) it is clear that the rates of shear to which blood is normally exposed *in vivo* or *in vitro* should have an im-measurable effect upon the viscosity of solutions of the plasma proteins. This was confirmed by Wells et al. (1964) who reported that solutions of fibrinogen were Newtonian even at concentrations of more than three times those found in normal plasma. It is also of interest to note that serum (which possesses no fibrinogen) has been classified as non-Newtonian (Kreuzer, 1950) although recent experiments have not confirmed this (Merrill *et al.*, 1963a; Chien *et al.*, 1966). Burgman *et al.* (1964) have suggested that plasma should be treated as a crystalline system whose rheological properties are determined by the density, generation, concentration and propagation of dislocations stemming from defects in the system. Thus in some cases it could deform plastically, like a normal crystalline system, leading to a definite yield stress; in others where the structural order was already broken down it could deform at all stresses and a yield stress would be absent. A difficulty with this theory is that there have been no experimental reports of plasma exhibiting a yield stress.

It should not be overlooked that some of the discrepancies which have been reported may have been due to uncertainties in the viscometry techniques used, including denaturing of the plasma at its interface with air or a protective fluid where it was used (Criddle, 1960; Merrill *et al.*, 1961, 1963a; Joly, 1965). But although they might lead to a Newtonian fluid exhibiting a shear-rate dependent viscosity it is extremely unlikely that instrument defects would cause the opposite effect and it is possible that some of the viscometers have been insufficiently sensitive to detect any deviations from Newtonian behaviour which were, in fact, present. They are undoubtedly small when compared with those exhibited by whole blood and suspensions of red cells (see Chapter 6) and become insignificant at shear rates exceeding about 100 sec^{-1}. Even at low rates of shear when the effects are most marked the quoted deviations from Newtonian behaviour are so small that it is difficult to categorize plasma with complete certainty. Shorthouse *et al.* (1967) considered that sheep plasma behaved as a Maxwell fluid (p. 8) but numbers of investigators (Madow *et al.*, 1956; Charm *et al.*, 1962; Bugliarello *et al.*, 1965) have shown that it corresponds reasonably well to a power-law fluid, the exponent s [eqn. (1.4)] lying between 0·95 and 0·995. This should be compared with a value of 1 given by Newtonian fluids and approximately 0·75 by suspensions of red cells.

Temperature

The viscosity of most fluids is sensitive to changes in temperature, and plasma is no exception. A fall of 2–3 per cent per °C rise in temperature has been reported in the temperature range 25–37°C (Merrill *et al.*, 1963a) which is similar to the temperature coefficient of whole blood (Green, 1944; Mayer *et al.*, 1965). A decrease in the temperature of a solution should lead to a reduction in the thermal energy of the system and to an increase in the alignment of asymmetric molecules at a given rate of shear. This might show as a reduction in the non-Newtonian behaviour of plasma with a reduction in temperature but it is probably immeasurable, even for the fibrinogen molecules which are the ones most likely to be affected in normal plasma. Merrill *et al.* (1963a) reported that normal human plasma was Newtonian at 37°C and 25°C, but Rand *et al.* (1964a) found that although human plasma was almost Newtonian at 37°C it became quite strongly non-Newtonian below 27°C.

Lipids

Lipids are often present in plasma in the form of a stabilized fat emulsion, the particles (or chylomicra) being some $0 \cdot 2$–$0 \cdot 5 \, \mu$ in diameter. It might be anticipated that an increase in the lipid content of the plasma would raise the viscosity but the quantity which can be absorbed is quite small (up to $0 \cdot 005$ g/ml) and is on the threshold of detection in existing viscometers so that no consistent measurable change has been reported (Charm *et al.*, 1963; Merrill *et al.*, 1964). The lipids probably influence to a limited extent the rheology of whole blood under some circumstances by aggregating the red cells although this property has not been fully confirmed by experiment (Swank, 1954, 1956, 1959).

CHAPTER 6

RHEOLOGY OF BLOOD

BEFORE considering the behaviour of blood when moving through vessels of various dimensions and geometries it is necessary to examine its bulk flow properties. Blood can be treated as a homogeneous fluid if the volume of the sample being sheared is large compared with the size of the red cells but if this is not feasible the possibility that interaction effects between the red cells and the containing surfaces are present must be considered and suitable corrections applied when necessary. Unfortunately it is frequently very difficult to decide whether or not such effects have influenced any measurements taken in a particular type of viscometer. In addition unknown edge effects may occur at the boundary to the sheared blood, affecting the flow pattern and possibly influencing the measured rate of shear.

In practice various compromises have to be made in the measurement. A large volume of blood is frequently difficult to obtain and, if available, there are problems in maintaining it at a constant temperature. Moreover, if the containing surfaces are situated far apart (compared with the size of the red cells) the forces present become extremely small and difficult to measure under streamline flow conditions. The characteristics of the different types of viscometers which have been used on blood were considered in Chapter 4; all have their advantages and disadvantages and at present no one type can be said to be best for measurements under all conditions. The bulk of the recent work on the rheology of blood has been carried out in cone plate and co-axial cylinder viscometers because the rate of shear is known with fair precision in these instruments and concentration changes often associated with tube viscometers (Chapter 8) are avoided. Blood is a complex heterogeneous system and although there is general agreement on some facets of its behaviour under shear, there are many on which no clear concensus of opinion has yet been reached.

The proportion of white cells and platelets present in whole blood is so small that it is unlikely that their presence makes a measurable change in the viscosity level. If plasma is Newtonian in its behaviour (or almost so) the viscosity of whole blood and of suspensions of red cells in natural plasma, serum and isotonic solutions, relative to the suspending medium η_r (p. 12) should be identical provided that the medium is always of about the same density and does not affect the flexibility or aggregation of the cells. However, there is evidence (Merrill *et al.*, 1963a, 1965b; Wells *et al.*, 1964; Chien *et al.*, 1966) that the proteins in whole blood may affect the aggregation of the cells so that it is more satisfactory to consider whole blood separately from suspensions of cells in other fluids.

Whole Blood

As soon as a blood sample is removed from a living animal the clotting mechanism comes into action and the viscosity of the blood steadily changes. It is usual, therefore, to add an anticoagulant which in some cases may dilute, or in other ways alter, the flow characteristics of the plasma; the findings of various workers were considered in Chapter 5. Some investigators have reported that the presence of an anticoagulant alters the viscosity of blood (Copley, 1960; Gelin, 1965), but recent experiments by Mayer *et al.* (1965) lead to the conclusion that the treatment of whole blood with heparin, sequestrene or oxalate makes no significant difference to its behaviour other than producing a simple diluting effect if the anticoagulant is in aqueous solution.

Flow-curve Characteristics

The basic shear stress/rate of shear characteristics of blood can be obtained without difficulty from cone plate or co-axial cylinder viscometry by the various techniques mentioned in Chapter 4. The flow curves obtained from different samples at the same haematocrit are difficult to compare, however, because it is not obvious to what extent the viscosity of the plasma (which may vary significantly from sample to sample) influences the results. It is more convenient to work in terms of the behaviour of blood relative to that of the plasma at the same rate of shear by plotting shear stress, corrected to a plasma viscosity of unity τ/η_o against the rate of shear D. The slope of a line drawn from any point on the curve to the origin is then equal to the apparent viscosity of the blood (relative to the plasma) at the selected rate of shear. Unfortunately not all workers have given sufficient information for their results to be plotted in this way but the available data are included in Fig. 6.1. They strongly suggest non-Newtonian behaviour, particularly at

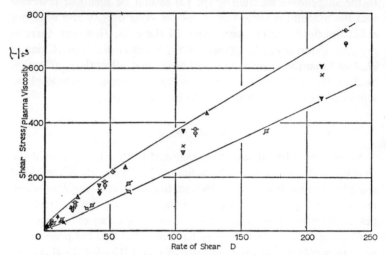

FIG. 6.1. Flow curve for human blood and red cells suspended in plasma (shear stresses are adjusted to a plasma viscosity of unity).

Key:	Symbol	Reference	Temp. (°C)	Haematocrit %
	⊡	Bugliarello et al., (1963)	30	40
	⊡	Bugliarello et al., (1965)	29	37·5
	◇	Chien et al., (1966)	37	45
	▽	Gelin (1965)	37	44
	-○-	Groth (1966) Men	37	Normal
	○	Groth (1966) Women	37	Normal
	▲	Merrill et al., (1961)	37	43
	△	Merrill et al., (1963a)	37	42·5
	×	Rand et al., (1964a)	37	40

Units: Ordinate, Abscissa; sec⁻¹.

low rates of shear, and it is now necessary to examine the validity of the various equations which have been proposed for describing the flow characteristics of blood.

Power Law. We can test whether whole human blood or human cells resuspended in plasma behave as a power-law fluid by plotting $\log \tau/n_\theta$ against $\log D$ for the data from different workers when using rotating viscometers (Fig. 6.2). It will be observed that the points lie in a broad band which shows distinct curvature but no obvious distinction between whole blood and resuspended cells in plasma. Thus power-law behaviour, which would be represented by a straight line, is not confirmed although over small ranges of shear rate it might be accepted as an approximation. Values of the exponent s [eqn. (1.4)] of $0.68-0.80$ which have been suggested by various workers (Charm et al., 1962; Bugliarello et al., 1963, 1965;

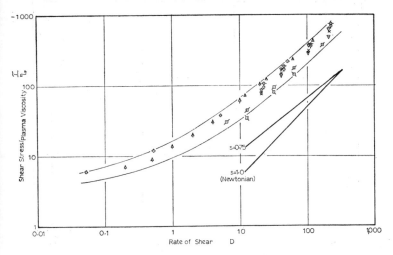

FIG. 6.2. Flow curve for human blood and red cells resuspended in plasma, plotted on logarithmic scales (shear stresses are adjusted to a plasma viscosity of unity).

Key: As given for Fig. 6.1.
Units: Ordinate, Abscissa; sec^{-1}.

Hershey et al., 1966) using rotating viscometers are therefore not unreasonable in the range of shear rates between about 5 and 200 sec^{-1}. The value of s may be influenced by the type of instrument used because Madow et al. (1956), Charm et al. (1962) and Hershey et al. (1966) obtained values of s which, for human, canine and human blood respectively, were greater than 0.9 when measured in tube viscometers. The mean rates of shear were a little greater in the tube instruments than the rotating viscometers but it is uncertain whether this factor alone explains the appreciable difference in shear-rate dependence observed in the two instruments.

Bingham Plastic. Figure 6.1 suggests that although blood may behave as a Bingham plastic it does not follow the flow curve for the idealized material [Fig. 1.6 and eqn. (1.7)]. In Fig. 6.3 its correspondence to the Casson equation [eqn. (1.8)] has been tested by plotting $\sqrt{(\tau/\eta_o)}$ against $\sqrt{D}$. The method of least squares gives the following equation of best fit.

$$\sqrt{\left(\frac{\tau}{\eta_o}\right)} = 1\cdot53\ \sqrt{D} + 2\cdot0. \qquad (6.1)$$

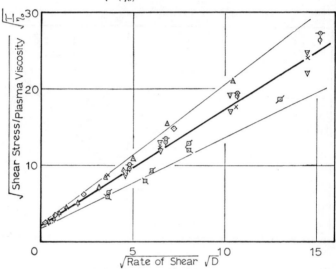

FIG. 6.3. Flow curve for human blood plotted to test the Casson equation (shear stresses are adjusted to a plasma viscosity of unity).

Key: As given in Fig. 6.1.

Units: Ordinate, Abscissa; $\sec^{-\frac{1}{2}}$.

TABLE 6.1

Viscosity of normal human blood

Investigator	Men (poise)	Women (poise)	Rate of shear ($\sec^{-1}$)
Rosenblatt *et al.* (1965)	0·0365–0·0553	0·0301–0·0489	230
Groth (1966)	0·0437–0·0457	0·0410–0·0428	230
Charm *et al.* (1965)	0·035		230
Equation (6.1)†	0·033		230

†Assuming a plasma viscosity of 0·012 poise.

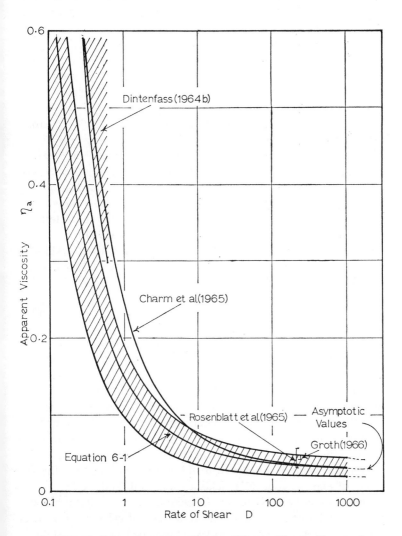

FIG. 6.4. Variation of apparent viscosity of human blood with rate of shear [eqn. (6.1) is plotted on the assumption that the viscosity of plasma is 0·012 poise].
Units: Ordinate; poise, Abscissa; sec⁻¹.

Assuming a plasma viscosity of 0·012 poise (Chapter 5) the mean viscosity of human blood at various rates of shear is then as given in Table 6.1 and Fig. 6.4.

Charm *et al.* (1965) have fitted Casson equations directly to samples from a blood bank without making allowances for differences in plasma viscosity. Satisfactory fits were obtained for shear rates between 0 and 100,000 sec^{-1}, the averaged equation being

$$\sqrt{\tau} = 0 \cdot 166 \sqrt{D} + 0 \cdot 33. \tag{6.2}$$

The viscosity of human blood at a shear rate of 230 sec^{-1}, as obtained from eqn. (6.2) is compared with values obtained by other experimenters in Table 6.1 and Fig. 6.4. Equation (6.2) after transposing to apparent viscosity/rate of shear coordinates is also shown graphically in Fig. 6.4 together with limiting values of the characteristics of normal human blood as proposed by Dintenfass (1964b).

Cokelet *et al.* (1963) reported that normal blood always exhibited a yield stress. At haematocrits exceeding 5–8 per cent Merrill *et al.* (1963b, 1964) found that the value was given by

$$\tau_y{}^{1/3} = A \, (H - H_m)/100 \tag{6.3}$$

where $A = (0 \cdot 008 \pm 0 \cdot 002 \text{ dyne/cm}^2)^{\frac{1}{3}}$, $H =$ normal haematocrit, and $H_m =$ haematocrit below which there is no yield stress. It may be noted that eqn. (6.3) is a special case of eqn. (1.12). Taking the haematocrit as 45 per cent, and H_m as 5 per cent, the yield stress of normal human blood should lie between 0·01 and 0·06 dyne/cm^2. Merrill *et al.* (1965a) reported good agreement with this conclusion from measurements in tube viscometers. Charm *et al.* (1965) found values ranging from zero to 0·14 dyne/cm^2, depending upon the viscometer, while if a value of 0·012 poise is assumed for the viscosity of plasma, eqn. (6.1) yields a value of 0·05 dyne/cm^2.

On the other hand, Chien *et al.* (1966) have shown that if blood is sheared at lower and lower rates in a co-axial cylinder viscometer ever-increasing apparent viscosities are recorded and they cast doubt on the existence of a yield stress. This difference in conclusion could be due to misapprenhensions concerning the behaviour of Bingham plastics in a rotating viscometer which must now be considered.

The concept of yield stress (or yield point) was originally developed for solids and it defines the stress at which irreversible physical changes occur in a body. In contrast, the internal structure of a Bingham plastic is not permanently destroyed by shearing and the planes of shear heal themselves on standing so that the yield stress does not correspond to a point of irreversible change in the material. A Bingham plastic will always flow in a rotating viscometer if the stress is allowed to rise sufficiently although the shearing will not normally be uniform throughout the material at low shear rates, even in a cone-plate viscometer (Boardman *et al.*, 1963). This can lead to a flow curve which exhibits no yield stress even though other instruments may prove its presence. Wells *et al.* (1964) found an abrupt change in the shear stress/rate of shear characteristic of whole human blood at a shear rate of about 1 sec^{-1}; this might well correspond to such a change in the shearing pattern in the blood sample. Rotating viscometers are fundamentally unsuited to yield stress measurements unless they can operate under conditions of constant stress because they are unable to detect directly the disruptive stress of any static structure which is present. A different type of instrument is more satisfactory for this type of measurement (Boardman *et al.*, 1961).

There is no doubt that any yield stress which is present in normal human blood is extremely small, probably less than $0 \cdot 1$ dyne/cm^2. But it could affect significantly the velocity profile and pressure drop in a narrow tube at low velocities of flow. For example, if a value of $0 \cdot 035$ poise is assumed for the viscosity of blood, the mean flow velocity in a tube $200 \, \mu$ in diameter for a pressure gradient of $0 \cdot 3$ cm of water per cm length of tube will be 1 mm/sec [from eqn. (3.5)]. The mean rate of shear in the blood will then be about 30 sec^{-1} [from eqns. (3.7) and (3.8)]. If, however, the blood possesses a yield stress of $0 \cdot 05$ dyne/cm^2 in addition to a viscosity of $0 \cdot 035$ poise at high rates of shear, the quantity flowing down the tube with the same pressure gradient will be reduced by almost 40 per cent [eqn. (3.16)]. Thus the assumption of Newtonian behaviour is most likely to lead to errors in the microcirculation or under any pathological conditions which greatly reduce the flow rate; these aspects are considered in later chapters.

At high rates of shear the non-Newtonian characteristics of blood become insignificant and may in most cases be ignored. The point of changeover cannot be specified with precision and depends on a variety of factors, including the haematocrit, but the data in Fig. 6.4 support the conclusion reached elsewhere (Whitmore, 1963,

1965a) that above shear rates of 50–100 sec^{-1} the apparent viscosity of a given blood sample is practically constant.

Haematocrit

Normal bloods generally possess haematocrits of 40–45 per cent so that experiments to relate viscosity to haematocrit are usually made on artificially prepared samples. The procedure is to separate the cells from the plasma by centrifugation and then to remix cells and plasma in the desired proportions, after removing the "buffy coat" of leucocytes and platelets.

Although it might be expected that the viscosity of whole blood from a particular species should increase with increasing haematocrit (see Chapter 1) it was shown above that the actual value at a given haematocrit depends upon the rate of shear chosen for the measurements. Thus if comparative measurements are made in a tube viscometer subjected to a constant pressure difference across its ends the flow rate will decrease as the haematocrit rises leading to a fall in the mean rate of shear and a rise in the measured viscosity, unless all the measurements are made at very high flow rate.

Examination of the available rotating-viscometer data (Rand *et al.*, 1964a, Bugliarello *et al.*, 1965, Chien *et al.*, 1966) suggests that the non-Newtonian behaviour of blood (as shown by the extent to which *s* in eqn. (1.4) differs from unity) increases rapidly when the haematocrit rises above 20 per cent, possibly reaching a maximum at between 40 and 70 per cent. Chien *et al.* (1966) attributed the decay at high haematocrit to a changeover in the blood from a predominantly cell–protein to a cell–cell interaction but physical interference with the flexing movement of cells must undoubtedly play an important part.

Various authors have claimed linearity between haematocrit and the logarithm of the viscosity, and there is some theoretical justification for the suitability of such a relationship (Richardson, 1950). It has been confirmed by different workers (Haynes, 1960; Peric, 1963; Gregerson *et al.*, 1965; Chien *et al.*, 1966) using human blood at 37°C and approximately equal shear rates (Fig. 6.5). The constant of proportionality falls with increasing shear rate, the results of Rand *et al.* (1964a) at a higher rate of shear being included in Fig. 6.5 in order to show the effect. In contrast, suspensions of rigid, smooth, dispersed, equi-sized spheres (which are also included in

Fig. 6.5) show a concentration dependence which is better fitted by eqn. (4.1) and is not affected by the rate of shear unless concentrations of about 40 per cent are exceeded (Rutgers, 1962).

The viscosity of human blood is appreciably lower than that of a suspension of spheres at the same concentration, if the concentration

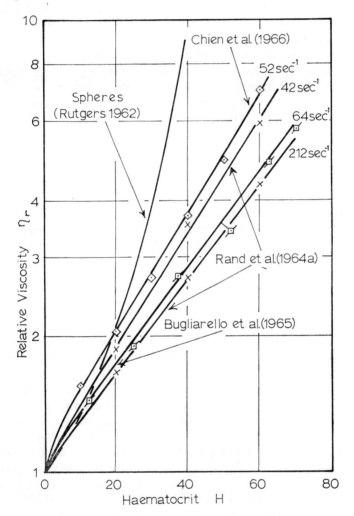

FIG. 6.5. Influence of haematocrit, on the relative viscosity of blood at various rates of shear.

Units: Abscissa; per cent.

exceeds about 10 per cent by volume (Fig. 6.5). Taylor *et al.* (1965) reported a tenfold difference over the shear rate range 0·1–100 sec^{-1} for concentrations of spheres corresponding to the normal haematocrit of blood. Because the viscosity of a suspension of dispersed spheres is independent of shear rate (at least up to concentrations of about 40 per cent) the lower viscosity exhibited by blood at haematocrits exceeding 10 per cent should become even more marked as the rate of shear is increased. In contrast the viscosity at low haematocrits appears to be higher for human blood cells than for spheres. The intrinsic viscosity [eqn. (1.9)] which equals 2·5 for suspensions of spheres is greater than 2·5 for blood and probably rises as the rate of shear is reduced, the results of Chien *et al.* (1966) showing an increase from 3·7 at 52 sec^{-1} to over 6·0 at 0·052 sec^{-1}.

Temperature

It is generally accepted that the temperature has very little effect on the relative viscosity of suspensions of rigid particles in simple liquids or on the yield stress when the suspension is flocculated (Goodeve, 1939; Rutgers, 1962). The work of Rothlin (Haynes *et al.*, 1959) demonstrated that the viscosity of blood, relative to water, rose as the temperature fell but this could have been because plasma is more temperature-dependent than water. Bugliarello *et al.* (1963) found that for a wide range of haematocrits the viscosity of human blood relative to plasma was not significantly different at temperatures ranging from 20 to 40°C. According to Azuma (1964), however, there was a 10 per cent rise in the relative viscosity of some bloods when the temperature was reduced from 37°C to 17°C which he attributed to a small increase in the volume of the individual cells together with an alteration in shape towards a more spherical and less disc-like form. There is no doubt that temperature can affect the physical properties of red cells (Teitel, 1965; Murphy, 1967) but Rand *et al.* (1964a) reported that the reduction of the temperature from 37°C to 22°C produced a fall in the relative viscosity of human blood of at least 15 per cent. Although these differences are not large it is clear that further work is required to clarify the influence of temperature on the flow properties of blood.

The effect of temperature on yield stress is also uncertain. Merrill *et al.* (1963b) concluded that it was generally unaltered by temperature in normal subjects but occasional increases have been reported when the temperature has been reduced.

Suspensions of Red Cells

The viscosity of human and other red cells when resuspended in a variety of media has been measured on a number of occasions. In the case of human cells the fluids include serum (Merrill *et al.*, 1963a; Chien *et al.*, 1966), albumin (Wells, 1965; Groth, 1966), globulin (Merrill *et al.*, 1965b; Wells, 1965), fibrinogen (Wells *et al.*, 1964; Merrill *et al.*, 1965b; Wells, 1965), saline (Wells *et al.*, 1964; Gelin *et al.*, 1965; Meiselman *et al.*, 1967; Wells, 1967), Ringers solution† (Merrill *et al.*, 1963a, 1965a; Chien *et al.*, 1966), ACD (Haynes *et al.*, 1959) and dextran (Gelin, 1965; Gelin *et al.*, 1965; Groth, 1966; Meiselman *et al.*, 1967; Wells, 1967). Not all suspending solutions were reported as showing Newtonian behaviour but deviations were usually less than 15 per cent over the range of shear rates used. An exception was high molecular weight dextran (Gelin, 1965) which showed pronounced non-Newtonian properties. In attempting to compare the results it must be borne in mind that the method of preparation of the suspensions almost certainly varied from worker to worker but a number of important conclusions, common to all the experiments, can be reached.

Plasma Constituents

Serum. Figure 6.6 shows that in contrast to whole blood, suspensions of red cells in serum follow a power-law relationship (eqn. 1.4) between shear stress and rate of shear over the range which has been tested. There is no evidence of the presence of a measurable yield stress and the results are fitted by the following equation

$$\tau = 10\eta_o \, D^{0.75}. \tag{6.4}$$

Data from tube viscometers on canine (Bayliss, 1960) and bovine (Müller, 1948; Kümin, 1949) cells in serum show somewhat similar behaviour but (as in the case of whole blood) the value of s is rather larger than in a rotating instrument and the shear rates are known

†Ringers solution normally consists of NaCl $0\cdot9$ g/100 ml, KCl $0\cdot42$ g/100 ml, $CaCl_2$ $0\cdot42$ g/100 ml, $NaHCO_3$ $0\cdot02$ g/100 ml.

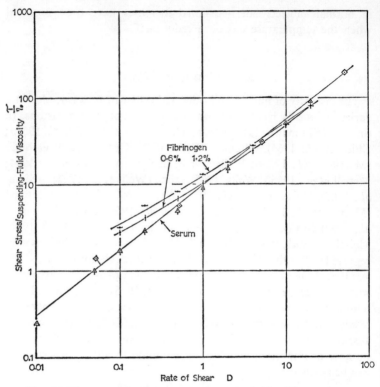

FIG. 6.6. Flow curves for human red cells suspended in different plasma constituents plotted on logarithmic scales (shear stresses are adjusted to a suspending fluid viscosity of unity).

Key:	Symbol	Reference	Temp. (°C)	Haematocrit (%)	Suspending fluid
	◊	Chien et al., (1966)	37	40	Serum
	△	Merrill et al., (1963a)	37	43	Serum
	─●─	Wells et al., (1964)	37	40	0·6% Fibrinogen
	⬥	Wells et al., (1964)	37	40	1·2% Fibrinogen

Units: Ordinate, Abscissa; sec^{-1}.

less precisely. At shear rates exceeding 1 sec^{-1} the non-Newtonian behaviour of suspensions of red cells in serum is rather similar to that of whole blood. Below this value the divergence which occurs is believed to be due to the absence of fibrinogen which leads to the disappearance of the yield stress (Merrill et al., 1963a).

Proteins. Wells (1965) has measured the viscosity of human red cells suspended in individual protein solutions of the type and at the concentration met with in normal human blood (Table 6.2).

ALBUMIN solutions do not aggregate human red cells (Wells, 1965; Merrill *et al.*, 1965b; Groth, 1966) and indeed they may promote the dispersion of rouleaux (see p. 85). The red cell suspensions do not exhibit a yield stress.

GLOBULINS raise appreciably the general viscosity level of plasma (and thus of whole blood) because they are present in high concentrations compared with the other proteins. They are reported to increase the rouleaux-forming abilities of the cells (Fahraeus, 1929), particularly when present in the β form but this does not lead to the development of a measurable yield stress unless fibrinogen is also present (Merrill *et al.*, 1965b). A remarkable feature reported by Wells (1965) is that human red cells suspended in globulin solutions of normal physiological concentration exhibited a higher viscosity at all rates of shear than whole blood (Table 6.2).

TABLE 6.2

Apparent viscosity of red cells suspended in protein fractions[1]

Temperature 37°C   Haematocrit 49 per cent

Suspension	Protein concentration (g/100 ml)	Apparent viscosity† (poise)
Whole human blood	Normal	0·076
Red cells in albumen	3·5	0·056
Red cells in globulin	2·2	0·106
Red cells in fibrinogen	0·6	0·042

[1] Wells (1965).   †Rate of shear 100 sec^{-1}

FIBRINOGEN solutions quickly aggregate red cells into rouleaux and form complete structures but large aggregates and rapid settlement appear only when the normal physiological concentration of 0·3 g/100 ml is exceeded (Wells *et al.*, 1964). However, Fig. 6.6 shows that even when 1·2 g/100 ml of fibrinogen was present the divergence of flow behaviour of human red cells at 40 per cent haematocrit from Newtonian or power-law behaviour was considerably less than that of whole blood (Fig. 6.2) so that some additional reagent to fibrinogen must be brought into play in whole plasma (Merrill *et al.*, 1966). For example, Copley *et al.* (1967) reported that the presence of minute quantities of fibrinogen–fibrin complexes led to a dramatic increase in the yield stress. Merrill *et al.* (1965b) found that when fibrinogen was present with other proteins in normal blood the yield stress τ_y was related to the fibrinogen concentration w_f by the equation

$$\tau_y = \frac{(H - 7)(1 \cdot 55\, w_f + 0 \cdot 76)^2}{100} \qquad (6.5)$$

when w_f is between $0 \cdot 21$ and $0 \cdot 46$ g/100 ml, and H is greater than 5–8 per cent.

Electrolytes

The logarithmic flow curves of suspensions of human cells in saline and Ringers solution at haematocrits of about 40 per cent as reported by various workers are shown in Fig. 6.7. They all fall on the same line, the linearity of whose slope suggests an absence of a yield stress. The angle of slope s is about $0 \cdot 9$ indicating appreciably more Newtonian behaviour than in the case of whole blood or red cells suspended in serum. Visual and viscometric measurements confirm an almost complete absence of aggregation of red cells when suspended in both liquids (Wells *et al.*, 1964; Merrill *et al.*, 1965b; Chien *et al.*, 1966).

Dextran

The therapeutic value of infusions of dextran has been recognized for many years (Bernstein *et al.*, 1960; Gelin, 1961; Groth *et al.*, 1964a; Ehrly, 1966; Groth, 1966) and the question of the extent to which the infusions alter the rheological properties of the blood is obviously important. *In vitro* tests on human cells in dextran solutions show that the degree of aggregation rises with molecular weight (when this exceeds about 30,000) and concentration, increasing the settling rate of the cells and the yield stress of the suspension (Thorsen *et al.*, 1950; Meiselman *et al.*, 1967).

The viscosities of dextran solutions at isotonic concentrations are appreciably greater than those of plasma and they increase the

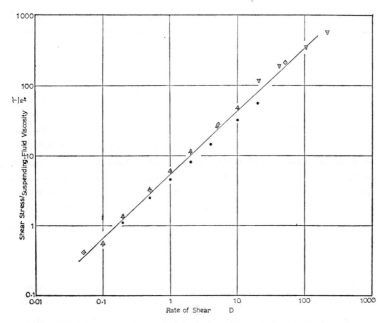

FIG. 6.7. Flow curves for red cells suspended in different solutions of
electrolytes, plotted on logarithmic scales (shear stresses are adjusted
to a suspended fluid viscosity of unity).

Key: Symbol	Reference	Temp. (°C)	Haematocrit (%)	Suspending fluid
◊	Chien *et al.*, (1966)	37	40	Ringers soln.
▽	Gelin (1965)	37	40	Saline soln.
△	Merrill *et al.*, (1963a)	25	43	Ringers soln.
●	Wells *et al.*, (1964)	37	40	Saline soln.

Units: Ordinate, Abscissa; sec^{-1}.

viscosity of treated blood (Groth *et al.*, 1965). The yield stress, which
presumably results from red cell aggregation (see Chapter 10),
also raises the measured viscosity but its importance decreases as
the rate of shear rises so that at shear rates exceeding about 20
sec^{-1} its contribution is insignificant (Gelin, 1965; Whitmore, 1967a).
On the other hand, the fall in haematocrit following dilution with
dextran solution slightly reduces the relative viscosity and the yield
stress. Figure 6.5 shows that a simple reduction in the haematocrit
of normal human blood by dilution from 45 to 40 per cent lowers the
relative viscosity at high rates of shear by about $12 \cdot 5$ per cent while
eqn. (6.3) shows that the yield stress falls by approximately 30

per cent. This causes the apparent viscosity to fall by at least 40 per cent at low rates of shear and by about 12·5 per cent at high. Present indications from *in vitro* experiments are that the addition of low molecular weight dextran to suspensions of red cells aggregated by fibrinogen or high molecular weight dextran does not lead to larger proportional falls in yield stress or viscosity than equal additions of saline or albumin solution (Ehrly, 1966; Meiselman *et al.*, 1967; Wells, 1967). In contrast, visual evidence from *in vitro* experiments is that the dispersion of red cells is increased by the addition of dextran solutions of 40,000 molecular weight at concentrations exceeding about 2 g/100 ml of blood, when compared with saline solution and dextran solutions of other molecular weights (Engeset *et al.*, 1966). Thus it appears that the relationship between aggregation (as assessed visually) and flow behaviour is not a simple one.

Haematocrit

The viscosity of a suspension of red cells is normally influenced by the rate of shear so that it is convenient to make comparisons at the same rates, or at rates which are so high that the asymptotic value of the viscosity is approached. Comparable information from different workers is unfortunately not always available but in Fig. 6.8 plots of the logarithm of the relative viscosity are made against haematocrit for suspensions of human cells in various suspending media when tested in rotating viscometers at approximately 50 sec^{-1}. A result at 212 sec^{-1} is also included to illustrate the influence of shear rate on the viscosity/haematocrit characteristics. The results can be compared with those for whole blood shown in Fig. 6.5 and the similarity is obvious after bearing in mind the differences between the suspending fluids employed, the experimental techniques used by the investigators and the designs of the instruments.

Measurements on human red cells suspended in ACD solution when made in tube viscometers (Haynes *et al.*, 1959) show similar characteristics to those obtained in rotating viscometers if the haematocrit exceeded about 20 per cent. At broadly comparable shear rates, however, the tube instrument gave slightly higher viscosities and this conclusion has been confirmed by Charm *et al.* (1962) on canine blood.

The rotating viscometer experiments lead to a value of more than 2.5 for the intrinsic viscosity [eqn. (1.9)] which is similar to the result

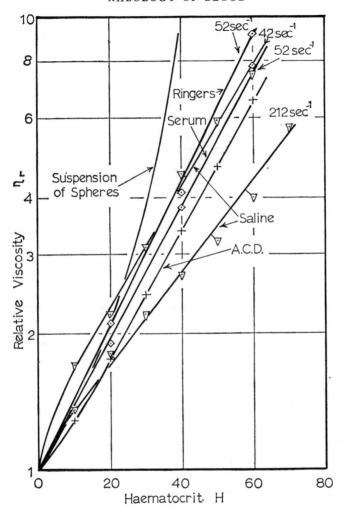

FIG. 6.8. Influence of haematocrit on the relative viscosity of suspensions of red cells in various media.

Key: Symbol	Reference	Temp. (°C)	Shear rate (sec^{-1})	Suspending fluid
◇	Chien *et al.*, (1966)	37	52	Ringers soln.
◈	Chien *et al.*, (1966)	37	52	Serum
▽	Gelin (1965)	37	42	Saline soln.
▽	Gelin (1965)	37	212	Saline soln.
+	Haynes *et al.*, (1959)	25·5	—	ACD soln.

Units: Abscissa; per cent.

obtained for whole human blood in similar instruments (see p. 72). On the other hand, the tube viscometer experiments lead to an intrinsic viscosity which is less than 2·5. The limited data available on other species of blood and red cell suspensions support the general conclusion that tube viscometry leads to intrinsic viscosities which are equal to or less than 2·5 (Whitmore, 1963). The disagreement with rotating viscometer results may be due to concentration changes which can occur when suspensions flow in narrow tubes at low concentrations and which are considered further in Chapter 8.

Influence of Cell Characteristics

Surface Charge

The flow characteristics of a suspension of particles are influenced by the degree of aggregation which is present. In the case of colloidal particles the surface charge is an important factor in determining the magnitude of the interparticle forces which control aggregation but Seaman (1967) found no change in the viscous properties of suspensions of human and canine cells when the surface charge was altered or completely removed (Seaman et al., 1965a). This may, in part, have been due to the comparatively high shear rates at which the measurements were made (11·5–230 sec^{-1}) but it is also possible that the volume of a red cell is so large that it should not be classed as a colloidal particle from the intercell attraction point of view.

Rigidity

The flexing of the red cells undoubtedly plays an important role in the shearing of blood. Seaman et al. (1967) found that canine cells in saline solution lost their non-Newtonian properties at haematocrits up to at least 40 per cent if they were hardened with aldehyde and this has been confirmed elsewhere (Gregerson et al., 1967). Moreover, their flow behaviour became more like that of dispersed spheres (Fig. 6.9) although in the haematocrit range of 20–30 per cent the viscosity level was similar to that of normal cells, confirming the observations of Kuroda et al. (1958).

Shape

Kuroda et al. (1958) found that the viscosity of suspensions of bovine cells which had been hardened after acquiring spherical shape was

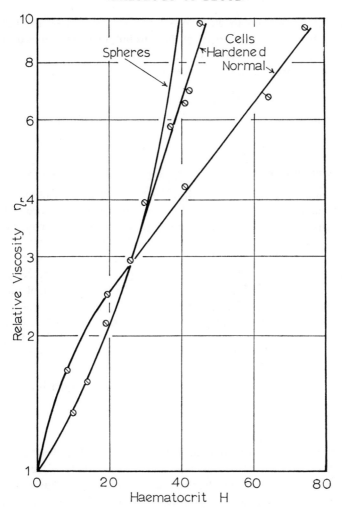

FIG. 6.9. Influence of haematocrit on the relative viscosity of normal and hardened cells suspended in saline solution (rate of shear 230 sec^{-1}).

Units: Abscissa; per cent.

appreciably higher than that of similar cells at the same haematocrit which had been hardened in their normal shape. Haematocrits of up to 75 per cent were used. Erslev *et al.* (1963) reported that there was a significant rise in the viscosity of whole blood when the mean concentration of haemoglobin in human red cells exceeded 34 per cent. It is uncertain to what extent this was caused by increased rigidity or increased sphericity of the cells but, in contrast to Kuroda *et al.* (1958), Seaman's results (1967) suggest that shape changes may have a relatively small influence on flow properties, spheres and hardened cells behaving very similarly except at high haematocrits (Fig. 6.9). Nevertheless, the shape is undoubtedly important in determining the amount of flexing which is possible in a non-rigid cell.

Size and Species

Strumia *et al.* (1963) found that if the mean volume of human red cells was within the range 58–117 μ^3 no significant difference in the viscosity could be detected while Gregerson *et al.* (1965) confirmed this conclusion from experiments on cells from different animal species which varied from 18 to 120 μ^3 in volume. This is understandable on the basis of all red cells behaving as smooth compact particles (Ward *et al.*, 1950) and deforming to a similar extent under similar conditions of shear. Conversely, Stone (1964) who also studied suspensions of red cells from different mammals found a distinct tendency for the viscosity to increase with decreasing size of the red cell at a given feed haematocrit but as his experiments were made in tube viscometers the haematocrits in the tubes may have been influenced by the size of the red cells (see Chapter 8).

Discussion

Over the last 60 years the flow behaviour of blood has been studied *in vitro* by many investigators who have used a variety of techniques and instruments. A considerable mass of information has accumulated but unfortunately a good deal of it is difficult to analyse or correlate because it is incomplete. Reviews of earlier data have appeared elsewhere (Bayliss, 1952; Scott Blair, 1958; Whitmore, 1963, 1965a) but one of the prime difficulties with experiments made before about 1960 is that they were carried out, almost without exception, in tube viscometers. These are cheap to build, easy to operate and their geometry corresponds roughly to that of a blood vessel in a living body. They suffer from the disadvantages of shearing the fluid at an inconstant rate and, in some cases, of producing haematocrit changes in the tube (see Chapter 8). Although blood is non-Newtonian the generalized method of handling tube viscometry data (described on pp. 54–5) can be used to obtain its basic flow properties if it is treated as a homogeneous fluid. Normally, however, insufficient data are available for this type of analysis to be made and the interpretation of the results becomes extremely difficult. Rotating viscometers give a nearer approximation to constant shear-rate conditions but suffer from the disadvantage of exposing an appreciable area of the blood to the air so that denaturing of the plasma may occur and affect the results. Moreover, if the instrument is designed to operate on small volumes of blood (which is a very desirable characteristic) the distance over which shear occurs is small, and corner (or end) effects may produce peculiar or unsuspected drag phenomena. Flow at low rates of shear may be restricted to a narrow layer of liquid adjacent to the viscometer wall, particularly if the flow of the main mass of blood is inhibited by the presence of a yield stress, and grooving of the surface may become necessary in order to transmit the full shear stress to the blood. The calibration of an instrument with Newtonian liquids does not always obviate these difficulties and there is obviously room for more correlation work between different shearing-zone geometries.

Another factor hampering the analysis of the resistance of blood to flow is a lack of general acceptance of the flow properties of plasma. A very convenient measure of the influence of the suspended matter upon the flow behaviour of a simple two-phase system is the relative viscosity (see p. 12). In the case of whole blood the viscosity is taken relative to that of the plasma, both being measured at the same rate of shear, but a difficulty immediately presents itself. If, for example, the sample of blood possesses an haematocrit of 50 per cent the rate of shear of the plasma is, on average, at least twice as great as that to which the sample is nominally exposed. This is because shearing is predominantly confined to the plasma. In addition, a proportion of the plasma may be continuously immobilized by attachment to single cells or through physical interactions between cells, leading to a further increase in the effective rate of shear in the remainder of the plasma. If the plasma is non-Newtonian and its apparent viscosity falls with increasing shear rate the contribution of the cells to the viscosity of blood (as measured by the relative viscosity) will always be underestimated. The difficulty is not avoided by considering the viscosity of blood in absolute terms or relative to water because the individual contributions of the plasma and the red cells to the total viscosity will be indeterminate.

Meaningful viscosity measurements on two-phase systems are recognized as difficult to make even when the system is rigidly defined. In the case of blood where innumerable subtle differences in the properties of the plasma and the cells may go undetected the problems are much greater. It is not surprising that reproducibility and correlation of experimental results are difficult to achieve but a number of important general conclusions may be drawn.

Rate of Shear. The flow behaviour of normal human blood (and indeed blood from all vertebrates which have been examined) depends upon the rate of shear to which it is exposed. The causes for this could reside in the flexibility of the cells, the presence of a yield stress, or both. The inherent flexibility of the red cells leads to their distortion when blood is sheared so that when flow ceases some relaxation should occur. But although there is a distinct possibility that blood should possess some visco-elastic properties, the few attempts which have been made to measure them have not been successful and calculations of relaxation times must be speculative until more is known of the elastic constant of the red cells. On the other hand, the hardening of the cells removes the non-Newtonian behaviour of blood (except at high haematocrits) and gives it the viscous properties of a suspension of compact, dispersed, rigid particles. The charge on the cells seems to have relatively little effect on the rheology of blood except at very low rates of shear, indicating that red cells should not be treated as colloidal particles.

Experiments strongly suggest that normal human blood possesses a small yield stress but the evidence is by no means conclusive. The presence of a yield stress in a suspension is normally conditional upon the constituent particles forming a connected structure which must be disrupted before continuous flow can commence. It represents the stress which is required to break the links in the structure and initiate motion. A prerequisite must therefore be the presence of a sufficient concentration of suspended matter to produce a structure and, in the case of blood, this is believed to correspond to an haematocrit of 5–8 per cent.

The primary aggregating agent in whole blood is claimed to be fibrinogen but it alone appears incapable of producing such a high yield stress as plasma even when present in large amounts. The relationship between aggregation and yield stress is unlikely to be a simple one because aggregation takes more than one form. In the most commonly reported type, two or more red cells form up in chains by contact between their discoidal surfaces to give rouleaux. It is not unreasonable to suppose that if red cells possess small attractive forces they move to positions of minimum energy (corresponding to the exposure of the minimum area to the plasma) and maximum mechanical stability which, for discoids, is the rouleau shape. Crenated mammalian cells and cells from some species (such as the frog) appear incapable of rouleau formation but they do not possess a bidiscoidal shape. Rigid spheres are incapable of forming rouleaux, possibly because of the mechanical instability of such a structure.

A second form is random aggregation, where the cells adhere to each other in no obvious structural pattern. Intermediate forms consisting of jumbled masses of small rouleaux are frequently observed and it is quite possible that the ultimate pattern is determined by the magnitude of the inter-cellular forces. If these are small, individual cells have the opportunity of moving into rouleaux while aggregating; if they are large and aggregation is rapid the cells become interlocked into larger masses before rouleau formation can commence. Red cell aggregation is an unimportant transient phenomenon in healthy mammals but it is an intrinsic feature of many pathological conditions and is considered again in Chapter 10 from that point of view.

The yield stress in normal human blood is less than $0 \cdot 1$ dyne/cm² which is remarkably small compared with those exhibited by, for example, suspensions of flocculated micron-size spheres at much lower volume concentrations. This suggests a form of attachment between red cell membranes which is not comparable with that between rigid surfaces.

Rheologically speaking, mammalian blood is best described as a Bingham plastic. The non-Newtonian characteristics of human blood probably reach a maximum at an haematocrit between 30 and 70 per cent and most of the experimental data on its flow properties are best fitted by the Casson equation [eqn. (1.8)]. An equation of the power-law type [eqn. (1.4)] is more satisfactory, however, for fully dispersed suspensions of red cells. It is important to note that the presence of the serum proteins appears to increase the non-Newtonian character of such suspensions without introducing a yield stress (compare Figs. 6.6 and 6.7). If the rate of shear exceeds about 100

sec^{-1} the non-Newtonian behaviour of mammalian blood at normal haematocrits becomes small and the relative viscosity settles down to a value between 3 and 4. This is less than one half of the value exhibited by suspensions of hard, smooth, equi-sized, dispersed spheres at the same concentration, the difference being primarily attributable to the flexibility of the red cells.

It is to be expected that the influence of cell flexibility on viscosity should diminish as the rate of shear is reduced and that the cells would behave as rigid bodies if the shear rate were made low enough. The flexing of the cells must absorb some energy particularly if they are visco-elastic but it could also reduce the volume of fluid immobilized during interactions, thus reducing the energy dissipation. Whether the net result would be an increase or a decrease in the bulk viscosity must depend upon the relative magnitudes of the cell flexure and cell interaction terms. The observed fall in apparent viscosity with increasing rate of shear suggests that at most haematocrits the interaction term falls faster than the flexure term rises as the shear rate is increased, and that suspensions of normal cells at high rates of shear should possess lower viscosities than suspensions of hardened cells. This is confirmed at medium or high haematocrits but at low haematocrits the position is not so clear. The intrinsic viscosity of a suspension records the influence of the dispersed phase when present in such low concentrations that interactions are unimportant. The results of Chien *et al.* (1966) show a rise in intrinsic viscosity with fall in rate of shear and it reached a value of about 6 at $0 \cdot 052$ sec^{-1}. This is much larger than the predicted figure of $3 \cdot 0$ for rigid oblate ellipsoids having about the same aspect ratio as blood cells (see Table 1.1) and Seaman (1967), *et al.* (1967) found that while hardened cells exhibited an intrinsic viscosity of $2 \cdot 5$ to 3, normal cells in the same rotating viscometer usually gave a higher value (Fig. 6.9). At low rates of shear an intrinsic viscosity in excess of 3 thus appears possible while at high shear rates it might fall to nearer $2 \cdot 5$ if the cells deformed into more compact shapes, but confirmatory experimental and theoretical work in this area is lacking. Tube viscometry leads to intrinsic viscosities of suspensions of red cells which are always equal to or less than $2 \cdot 5$ but these instruments are unsuitable for two-phase systems if the dispersed phase is present at low concentration because radial redistribution may take place and reduce the effective concentration. This problem is considered in more detail in Chapter 8.

Haematocrit. The relative viscosity of blood falls as the haematocrit is reduced until it reaches unity when red cells are completely absent. At high haematocrits it possesses a much lower viscosity than a suspension of smooth, rigid spheres of the same concentration but the difference falls with haematocrit and probably reverses at concentrations of less than 10 per cent, according to rotating-viscometer measurements.

Coagulation

If healthy blood is allowed to come into contact with surfaces outside normal living blood vessels it solidifies unless an anticoagulant is present. The result is the formation of a clot around any break in the vascular walls and coagulation (or clotting) in samples of blood removed from animals. *In vitro* experiments indicate that a clot consists predominantly of fibrin and red cells (Macfarlane, 1960; Biggs *et al.*, 1962). The fibrin is derived from the fibrinogen in the plasma by a complex chain of reactions, the normal clot owing its properties to the presence of fibrinogen, platelets, thrombin, calcium and serum; if one of these ingredients is deficient the rheology of the clot is altered (Hartert, 1960).

Under certain conditions clotting can occur intravascularly but the clots differ microscopically from those produced *in vitro* by including platelet masses (Rozenberg *et al.*, 1966) and their biological and physical properties are so difficult to measure that their rheology is virtually unknown. It is interesting to note that although the biochemistry of clotting is covered by an enormous literature (Biggs *et al.*, 1962) the rheological aspects have been neglected up to quite recently. This is not really surprising in view of the difficulty of making meaningful measurements.

The study of blood clotting is conveniently divided into three phases: first, changes in viscosity before any change in the appearance of the blood is observed, second the formation of a complete structure (or clot), and third, the contraction (or retraction) of the clot. The second phase has been divided by Copley *et al.* (1960) into two sub-stages.

The first phase has been examined by Dintenfass (1965b) who found that at body temperatures the rapidity of clotting increased with increasing rate of shear, the pattern being reversed at lower temperatures. The rate of shear also influenced the structure of the clot which was finally formed (Rozenberg *et al.*, 1964). Typical

times before a significant rise in the viscosity level of the blood occurred were 4 to 7 minutes but it is reported to be affected not only
by the health of the donor (Dintenfass, 1963a) but also by his psy-
chological state (Scott Blair, 1960).

Measurements are difficult to make during the subsequent stages
of clot formation and retraction. The system is not in equilibrium
and it is likely that the way in which the structure of fibrin strands
forms is influenced by the geometry of the system used and the shearing which the blood may undergo while measurements are being
made. The rheological properties of the forming clot are determined
chiefly by its structure and the stretching effect of the contracting
mechanism (Hartert, 1965). Contraction probably commences as
soon as clotting commences but it is not until after 30 minutes or so
of coagulation that the expulsion of the fluid serum which it contains is observed (Macfarlane, 1961). Scott Blair (1960) found that
after some 15 minutes of coagulation the clot took on the properties
of a Maxwell fluid (p. 8), the elasticity and viscosity moduli rising
continuously as the clot retracted to give ultimate values of elasticity
modulus approaching 10^4 dyne/cm^2 (assuming a Poisson's ratio of
$0 \cdot 5$) and a viscosity of over 10^6 poise (Scott Blair, 1960; Scott Blair
et al., 1960). Dintenfass (1963b) reported that the clotting time decreased with increasing rate of shear while Scott Blair (1960) found
that if the blood was tested very frequently during coagulation the
clotting process seemed to be a little slower than when fewer tests
were made. A rest between tests was apt to produce an abnormally
rapid further hardening and this was attributed to some kind of
thixotropy. The shrinkage during coagulation may be prevented by
adhesion of the clot to the container wall but, if it is free to move
away, contraction continues until its volume is reduced to about one
half the original. Platelet aggregates are not visible in the resulting
clot unless a certain rate of shear was exceeded during clotting
(Rozenberg et al., 1966).

If the red cells are removed before clotting commences the
phenomenon of pure contraction of the fibrinogen structure can be
studied, when shrinkage up to 95 per cent of the original volume
may occur unless the structure is restrained. The initial presence of
platelets is essential to the development of such strongly contracting
clots (Macfarlane, 1960; Leroux, 1965; Hartert, 1967) but intimate
contact between them and the fibrin does not occur unless the platelet membranes are ruptured (Erichson et al., 1966).

It will be appreciated that the schemes of coagulation which form the basis of most experimental and academic biochemical work on clotting are still greatly simplified compared with the physiological system (Macfarlane, 1960) and it is clear that the rheology of coagulation is at an even less advanced state. Nevertheless, rheological techniques may prove very useful in the future for following biochemical changes in the blood during clotting.

CHAPTER 7

THE DYNAMICS OF THE CIRCULATION

BOTH the systemic and pulmonary vascular systems can be divided into three main parts:

The arterial bed; a distributing system.
The microcirculation; a diffusing system.
The venous bed; a collecting system.

The mean pressure of the blood when it leaves the left ventricle of the heart is approximately 100 mm Hg in man; this has fallen to less than 10 mm Hg by the time it returns to the heart. In Fig. 7.1 the mean pressure and the pressure variation in the various vessels is shown and it will be observed that the greatest resistance to flow is experienced in the microcirculation, particularly in the arterioles. The estimated percentage of the initial systemic circulation pressure which is lost by the blood in flowing through the different parts of the vascular system is given in Table 7.1. In the pulmonary circula-

TABLE 7.1

Pressure gradient in the systemic system

Structure	Total pressure gradient %
Arteries	10[1]
Arterioles	40[2]–60[1]
Capillaries	15[1]–30[2]
Venules	8[2]–10[3]
Veins	15[1]

[1] McDonald (1960b).
[2] Merrill *et al.* (1961).
[3] Greenfield (1962).

90

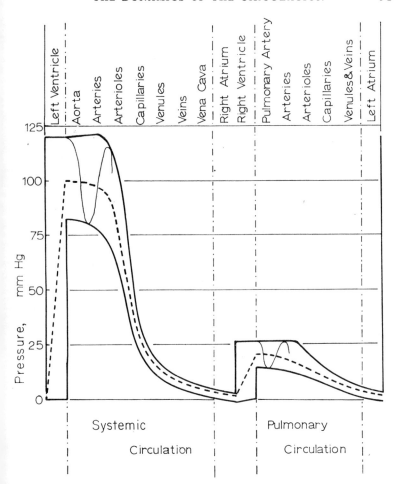

FIG. 7.1. Diagrammatic representation of the pressures and pressure variations in various parts of the circulation of man.

tion the absolute pressure level is considerably less than in the systemic circulation but again the pressure fall is primarily in the microcirculation.

Detailed measurements of the number and size of the blood vessels in living bodies are very difficult, time consuming and tedious to make and it is not surprising that reliable information is scarce. Moreover, it cannot be assumed that data collected on one tissue or

TABLE 7.2

Systemic circulation of a dog

Structure	Diameter (cm)	Number	Total cross-section area (cm^2)	Length (cm)	Total volume (cm^3)	Blood velocity (cm/sec)	Tube Reynolds number†
Aorta	1·0	1	0·8	40	30	50	1670
Large arteries	0·3	40	3·0	20	60	13	130
Main arterial branches	0·1	600	5·0	10	50	8	27
Terminal branches	0·06	1800	5·0	1	5	6	12
Arterioles	0·002	40 × 10^6	125	0·2	25	0·3	0·02
Capillaries	0·0008	12 × 10^8	600	0·1	60	0·07	0·002
Venules	0·003	80 × 10^6	570	0·2	110	0·07	0·007
Terminal veins	0·15	1800	30	1	30	1·3	6·5
Main venous branches	0·24	600	27	10	270	1·5	12
Large veins	0·6	40	11	20	220	3·6	72
Vena cava	1·25	1	1·2	40	50	33·0	1375

† Assuming viscosity of blood is 0·03 poise.

organ are applicable to another but some aggregate figures for dogs based by Green (1944) on Mall's original measurements (1888) are given in Table 7.2 because they are often quoted in the literature. Dimensional values should be considered only as relative but they indicate that some 30 per cent of the total blood volume is held in vessels smaller than about 1500 μ in diameter. On the other hand, it has been reported that about 80 per cent of the space enclosed by the vascular system of the rat contains vessels less than 188 μ in diameter (Knisely et al., 1958) and 88 per cent are smaller than 700 μ (Alexander, 1963). Apparent discrepancies in the distribution of blood between vessels of different sizes in the vascular system can probably be attributed to the specification of different size parameters in each case and to the variable capacity of the venous section.

The velocity of flow of blood in the circulating system ranges from more than 10 cm/sec in the arteries to less than 1 mm/sec in the capillaries, corresponding to an increase in the total cross-sectional area of the vessels between the aorta and the capillaries of at least 1000. Approximate values for flow velocities in the various parts of the vascular system of the dog are included in Table 7.2, together with the corresponding tube Reynolds numbers, assuming a value for the viscosity of the blood of 0·03 poise. Some comparable values for the circulating system of man are shown in Table 7.3 but in this case a viscosity of 0·035 poise is assumed for the calculation of Reynolds numbers.

TABLE 7.3

Systemic circulation of man

Structure	Diameter (cm)	Blood velocity (cm/sec)	Tube Reynolds† number
Ascending aorta	2·0[1]–3·2[2]	63‡[1]	3600–5800
Descending aorta	1·6[1]–2·0[2]	27‡[1]	1200–1500
Large arteries	0·2[1]–0·6[1]	20–50‡[1]	110–850
Capillaries	0·0005[3]–0·001[3]	0·05–0·1§[3]	0·0007–0·003
Large veins	0·5[3]–1·0[3]	15–20§[5]	210–570
Venae cavae	2·0[4]	11–16§[4]	630–900

[1] Spencer et al. (1963).   [3] Maggio (1965).
[2] Peterson et al. (1960).   [5] Brecher (1956).
[4] Helps et al. (1954).
† Assuming viscosity of blood is 0·035 poise.   ‡ Mean peak value.
§ Mean velocity over indefinite period of time.

The Arterial System

The outstanding feature of arterial blood flow is its pulsatile character. The sudden ejection of blood into the aorta from the left ventricle of the heart produces a wave of increased pressure and a slight distension of the arteries which change their diameter over the pressure cycle by less than 5 or 6 per cent of the mean value (Mc-Donald, 1960b; Peterson, 1962) because of their unusual rheological properties (Chapter 2). Between each stroke the arteries contract, maintaining the flow of blood although at a reduced rate. Because some muscular arteries contain a large mass of smooth muscle in their walls, the concept that they contract rhythmically with each heart beat and actively aid the flow has been put forward (Roston, 1964; Mitchell et al., 1965) but not substantiated (Rudinger, 1966).

A pressure wave is propagated along the arteries with each ejection of blood and is felt and recorded as the pulse beat. The velocity of propagation down the arterial tree is 10 to 20 times greater than the velocity of the blood and varies with the thickness and elasticity of the arterial wall (McDonald, 1960b). Arteries tend to become more rigid with advancing years and this is generally considered to be the cause of the increase in pulse velocity from an average rate of about 520 cm/sec at 5 years of age to 860 cm/sec at 84 (Winton et al., 1962). It is also very likely that the pulse velocity increases as it passes through the system, typical values being 500 cm/sec in the aorta and 800 or 1000 cm/sec in other arteries (Mc-Donald, 1960b).

As the pressure and flow-velocity pulses travel through the systemic system their profiles change (McDonald, 1960b; Mitchell et al., 1965) (Fig. 7.2), the amplitude of the flow pulse markedly decreasing and its width increasing with less back flow. This is the expected behaviour of waves propagated in viscous media where the effects of damping become important. But the transmission of the pressure pulse is accompanied by an increase in amplitude, usually combined with the development of a secondary oscillation (McDonald, 1960b). It has been attributed to the combined effects of reflection from points in the vascular tree (McDonald, 1960b; Attinger, 1963), the decreasing elasticity of the artery walls with increasing distance from the heart (Taylor, 1964), an increased arterial impedance towards frequencies above 10 c/s (Spencer et al., 1963) and resonance effects (Taylor, 1966a). The pattern of ejection from the right ventricle differs in detail from that of the left and the absolute pressure level is less but the behaviour of the pressure and flow pulses is similar in the systemic and pulmonary systems (Attinger, 1964a).

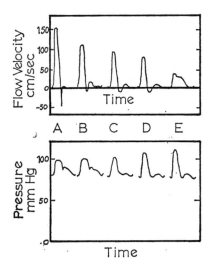

FIG. 7.2. Profiles of the flow velocity and pressure pulses in the peripheral arteries (after McDonald, 1960b).

A. Ascending aorta.
B. Thoracic artery.
C. Abdominal artery.
D. Femoral artery.
E. Saphenous artery.

Rheological interest in the arterial system centres on the extent to which the non-Newtonian properties of blood and the visco-elastic behaviour of the walls of the vessels influence flow resistance and pressure wave propagation in the system. This may depend upon whether the flow is laminar or turbulent.

Flow Behaviour

If the flow is laminar and steady, the rate of shear of a fluid flowing down a tube increases from zero at the axis to a maximum at the wall (see Chapter 3). Unsteady flow may modify this behaviour, giving a re-entrant velocity profile at certain periods of the cycle and increasing the mean rate of shear. But taking the steady-flow case and assuming a parabolic velocity profile, the data in Tables 7.2 and 7.3 lead to values for the rate of shear in the circulating system which are summarized in Table 7.4. It would seem that in the largest vessels the mean rate of shear is about 100–200 sec^{-1} and

TABLE 7.4

Rates of shear in the circulation[†]

Structure	Man		Dog	
	At the wall (sec^{-1})	Mean (sec^{-1})	At the wall (sec^{-1})	Mean (sec^{-1})
Ascending aorta	190[‡]	130 ⎫	400	270
Descending aorta	120	80 ⎭		
Large arteries	700	470	600	400
Capillaries	800	530	700	450
Large veins	200	130	50	35
Venae cavae	60	40	200	140

[†] Assuming parabolic velocity profile.
[‡] At peak velocity of flow.

reference to Fig. 6.4 (see p. 67) shows that the apparent viscosity of blood at these rates is some 10 per cent higher than the asymptotic value. If this is taken into account when calculating pressure gradients, energy losses and Reynolds numbers in the large vessels, the non-Newtonian properties of the blood can probably be ignored. On the other hand, if the flow in the vessels is turbulent it is evident from eqn. (3.10) (see p. 44) that the pressure gradient is approximately proportional to viscosity)$^{1/4}$. Thus in turbulent flow small variations in the viscosity, stemming from non-Newtonian behaviour, should have an insignificant effect upon the pressure gradient.

The patterns of flow which develop in the blood during its passage down the arteries are of considerable physiological significance (Mitchell *et al.*, 1965) and may be related to the onset of abnormalities and plaques in the vessel wall (see Chapter 10) but the difficulties of making direct observations of the interiors of intact arteries are very great because of the thickness of the walls. It has been usual to deduce whether the flow is laminar or turbulent from the ruling tube Reynolds number or from observations made on models. The amount of direct evidence is meagre and deductions from the tube Reynolds number or from flow in models have frequently been criticized. The lower critical Reynolds number for the appearance of stable turbulence in homogeneous liquids flowing at constant velocity along hard-walled cylindrical pipes is a little over 2000 (see p. 39) but the application of this parameter to the pulsating flow which is present in the arteries is undoubtedly questionable. Moreover, the condition for the transition back from turbulent to laminar flow is even more difficult to define in terms of a Reynolds number, particularly where eddies may be caused by a local disturbance (such as a junction) and would die out if sufficient distance of travel were available. The basing on Reynolds number criteria of the flow regime believed to prevail in the arteries and the larger veins must therefore be viewed with considerable suspicion but typical examples of mean values occurring in the vessels of dog and man are included in Tables 7.2 and 7.3 respectively.

Turbulence is most likely to occur in the aorta because the mean velocity is greatest there and the pulsatile nature of the flow should encourage it. Thus Timm (1942) found that the flow was laminar in the arched section of a model of a human aorta at a constant flow-rate but that it broke up into complex patterns in the following straight section. The mean velocity required for the development of turbulence appears to decrease with increasing pulse rate and Meisner et al. (1963) reported considerable turbulence in an aortic model under pulsatile flow conditions, particularly when the aortic valve was partially closed. On the other hand, Freis et al. (1964) found the flow in the ascending part of the aorta of a dog to be disturbed but not fully turbulent. The general consensus of opinion is that in the large arteries conditions for turbulence certainly occur, although the periods of high velocity are short and fully-developed turbulence may only occasionally be attained (McDonald, 1960a). But irrespective of whether the flow is laminar or turbulent, the non-Newtonian properties of the blood are probably relatively unimportant to flow resistance in the arterial tree. The small compensatory increase in apparent viscosity which is necessary if Newtonian behaviour is assumed reduces the effective Reynolds numbers in the vessels and slightly increases the calculated pressure gradient.

Attenuation

The factors controlling the transmission of the blood through the arterial system have been intensively studied and reviewed (McDonald, 1960a, b; Hardung, 1962; Spencer *et al.*, 1963; Attinger 1964b; Rudinger, 1966; Taylor, 1966a) and will not be discussed in detail here.

The velocity of propagation of the pressure wave in large arteries is insignificantly affected by the viscous components of the wall or the blood (Hardung, 1962; McDonald *et al.*, 1967), but in the attenuation which it suffers in transit the viscosity of the wall probably plays a more important role than that of the blood (Taylor, 1966a). It was deduced from a model consisting of randomly branching tubes that under conditions of propagation equivalent to those in a living body, a visco-elastic vessel wall attenuated the amplitude of an oscillation by more than 40 per cent after travelling one wavelength (Taylor, 1966b). Although the distance from the heart to the feet is only about a quarter of the wavelength of the fundamental component of the pressure pulse (McDonald, 1960b), the higher harmonics should be damped out quite quickly by the walls, contributing significantly to the change in the shape of the pressure wave as it travels through the arterial system (Fig. 7.2).

A major difference between constant and pulsatile flow is that the concept of resistance as embodied in the Poiseuille equation becomes inapplicable. A term must be found which describes the influence of the frequency of the oscillations on the relationship between the pressure and the flow rate. By analogy with the flow of an alternating current in an inductive or capacitative circuit the term *impedance* is often used (McDonald, 1960b; Taylor, 1966a). Its value is affected by the reflection of oscillations from the end of the system of tubes in which the measurements are made but it remains remarkably constant in the living arterial tree at all frequencies in excess of about 2 c/s (Taylor, 1966b). This is believed to be due to the combined effects of the elastic properties of the walls and the presence of many scattered terminations (Caro *et al.*, 1961). The relative contributions of the blood and the visco-elastic walls to the total energy dissipation cannot be calculated accurately (Peterson, 1962) but any dependence on the viscosity of the wall material or the blood is probably only slight (Taylor, 1966b). Attinger *et al.* (1967) and McDonald *et al.* (1967) found the attenuation in some arteries of dogs to be at least twice that calculated from Poiseuille's equation [eqn. (3.5)] but turbulence and curvature or tapering of the vessels may have contributed substantially to the extra pressure drop. Taylor (1966a) estimated that the extra work required by the left ventricle of the heart in performing pulsatile flow was only 5–15 per cent of that for constant flow. A variety of models has been suggested to simulate flow in the arterial system (see, for example: Wombersley, 1957; Lambert, 1958; Streeter et al., 1963; Rubinow et al., 1967; Seymour, 1967; Taylor, 1966b) but none can be said to give a really satisfactory representation of the in vivo situation as it is understood at present, except in general terms.

The Microcirculation

The microcirculation comprises a complex multiplicity of blood vessels ranging in diameter from about 30 cell diameters (in arterioles and venules) to less than one cell diameter in width (in the capillaries). Table 7.1 and Fig. 7.1 show that an important characteristic is that it is responsible for between three-quarters and four-fifths of the total pressure gradient in the vascular system (McDonald, 1960b; Merrill et al., 1961). The pulsatory characteristics of arterial blood have largely been damped out, although to a greater degree in the systemic than in the pulmonary system (Spencer et al., 1963; Wagner et al., 1963; Morkin et al., 1964), and the flow is sufficiently slow for the viscous properties of the blood to be extremely important. On the other hand, the virtual disappearance of the pressure wave greatly reduces the importance of the visco-elastic properties of the vessel walls. For example, Olson (1964) found that the vessels in a fully dilated limb behaved as rigid tubes after a certain pressure gradient was exceeded across the walls. Typical dimensions, pressure gradients and approximate flow rates in the various parts of the microcirculation are summarized in Fig. 7.1 and Tables 7.1, 7.2 and 7.3.

Flow Patterns

The particulate nature of blood becomes increasingly important in determining its flow properties as the diameter of the vessel diminishes. It can no longer be treated as a fluid because the red cells, which possess some degree of rigidity, are restricted in the orientations and positions which they can assume adjacent to the vessel wall.

The mean haematocrit is reduced in this area and a large proportion of the shearing during flow takes place in it (Macfarlane, 1961). Nevertheless, some relative motion between the cells in the main core also occurs at normal haematocrits and assumes two general forms. In the first, the cells arrange themselves in roughly concentric laminae with their discoidal surfaces oriented predominantly parallel to planes passing through the vessel axis. The centre core travels most rapidly, each additional layer passing more slowly than the one inside it (Knisely et al., 1950) and the leucocytes and platelets accompany the peripheral cells (Phibbs, 1966). The preferred orientation of the cells parallel to the tube axis has been confirmed by sectioning rapidly frozen blood vessels some 100 and 15 cell diameters in width taken from rabbits and dogs respectively (Phibbs, 1967; Wiederhielm et al., 1967). The degree of orientation of the cells increases with the flow rate (Bloch, 1966a) and although some cells may move in contact with the wall during flow (Phibbs, 1967), a plasma layer which on average is between a half and one cell diameter in width is present over a wide range of vessel diameters (Bloch, 1963). The thickness of the plasma region at the wall may also be velocity-dependent (Copley et al., 1962), disappearing when flow ceases (Bloch, 1963; Maggio, 1965). The orientation has been shown to account for the bright streak which is often seen down the axes of vessels conveying blood (Wiederhielm et al., 1967) and the flow pattern is frequently referred to as "laminar" (Maggio, 1965) although the term has a different physical significance in this context from when applied to pure fluids (see p. 37).

In the second pattern there is a random orientation of the red cells and every small portion of the blood mass oscillates across the tube in an irregular fashion, the cells bending, rotating, tumbling and exchanging places in a chaotic manner (Müller, 1948; Merrill et al., 1961; Maggio, 1965). They make frequent intimate contact with the walls, and plasma spaces not infrequently extend transversely across a third or more of the cross-section of the vessel (Bloch, 1963). This type of flow has been called "turbulent" (Maggio, 1965) and "Newtonian" (Müller, 1948), both terms unfortunately being liable to create confusion. The tube Reynolds numbers are so low that the flow is extremely unlikely to be truly turbulent (see p. 38) while "Newtonian" flow might well be thought to relate to the behaviour of a simple Newtonian fluid whereas blood in these small vessels exhibits much more complex properties.

THE DYNAMICS OF THE CIRCULATION 101

The extent to which it is valid to divide the blood flow patterns in vessels exceeding 8 or 10 cell diameters in width into two groups is uncertain. The rates of flow in healthy animals are so fast, even in small arterioles and venules, that at the magnifications required to observe individual cells their separate identification becomes impossible (Bloch, 1962, 1963). If the flow rate is reduced to a value where individual cells can be followed by eye, the interference which the system must suffer in making the reduction may inflict permanent damage upon it. But Block (1962, 1966a) has used a film speed of over 3000 frames/sec to show that in many preparations what to the eye appears as a homogeneous, laminar-flowing column of blood is, in fact, a tumbling mass of cellular components, and other observers have confirmed this (Merrill et al., 1961; Berman, 1964). It is clear therefore that photographic evidence of "laminar" flow from cine films taken at normal speed must be treated with some reserve. There is also the possibility that a constriction in a vessel or an asymmetry in the geometry of the wall may disturb the red cells and upset their orientation (Phibbs, 1967), while junctions or bends under some circumstances have a similar effect (Stehbens, 1967a). In both flow patterns, however, relative movement between the red cells in the core is a common factor and an appropriate name for the flow is "shearing-core" (Whitmore, 1967b). A subdivision can then be made between *oriented* shearing-core flow and *random* shearing-core flow to describe the two phenomena discussed above.

As the vessel size decreases from the larger arterioles and venules to the terminal arterioles and capillaries there is an imperceptible transition in the bulk flow pattern from shearing-core patterns, through the condition where the passage of one individual cell past another can only be achieved by deformation of both the bodies concerned, to the flow in the narrowest arterioles and capillaries where only single file progress is possible. Under these conditions an important characteristic of the flow is the variety of shapes which the red cells can assume. They may elongate or flex, sometimes symmetrically sometimes not, and rotate about an axis which forms an angle with the elongation and flection axes (Berman, 1964; Brånemark et al., 1963; Brånemark, 1965). When the diameter of the vessel approximates to the diameter of the cells the longest axis may be oriented in the direction of flow (Bloch, 1963) particularly if the cells are ellipsoidal. In contrast, discoidal shapes tend to move axially with their faces perpendicular to the direction of flow (Merrill et al.,

1961) either in short trains (Monro, 1963) or individually. They may deform into an unspecified number of shapes as they move (Bloch, 1963) while tear-drop (Monro, 1964), parabolic (Palmer, 1959; Guest *et al.*, 1963) and bullet (Stalker *et al.*, 1966) forms have been clearly distinguished. In all but the very smallest vessels the flexibility of the cells leads to the appearance of a thin layer of plasma at the wall (Brånemark, 1965). Because each cell practically fills the cross-section of the vessel along which it is moving the pattern has been called "plug" flow (Maggio, 1965). This term is unfortunate in that it is used in rheology to describe the behaviour of Bingham plastics in tubes at low flow velocities. An alternative which is preferred and is used here is "axial-train" flow (Whitmore, 1967b) (see Fig. 8.8).

It has been mentioned that whereas in axial-train flow the red cells have a preferred orientation with their discoidal surfaces perpendicular to the tube axis, in oriented shearing-core flow the tendency is for the discoidal surface to be parallel to the tube axis. Axial-train flow is observed in the narrowest vessels while oriented shearing-core flow occurs in vessels some cell diameters in width so that there must be a range of vessel diameters in which a transition from one form of cell orientation to the other takes place. It is possible that this intermediate region is typified by random shearing-core flow although this does not appear to have been investigated systematically.

Junctions

At diverging junctions in the microcirculation the concentrations of red cells in the two branches may differ considerably, not only because the concentration of cells in the feeding vessel may vary from instant to instant (Monro, 1963), but also because of *plasma skimming* (Krogh, 1922). This occurs when a minor vessel draws blood from a larger vessel in which there is a layer predominantly of plasma at the wall; the tendency is for the side vessel to draw a preponderance of plasma, the fluid being practically devoid of cells in some cases (Berman, 1963). It has been suggested that the presence of "cushions" or streamlined intrusions in the small arteries which surround some branch outlets encourages withdawal from the main flow rather than from the plasma wall layers (Fourman *et al.*, 1961) but visual evidence is that a plasma layer maintains its character past undulations in the vessel wall unless they are very abrupt (Maggio, 1965; Stehbens, 1967a). At narrow-angle, symmetrical, diverging junctions of small arteries or arterioles the bright streak which is often visible down the centre of the vessel (see p. 100) can be seen to split and re-centre in each outlet over a distance of 20 or 30 vessel diameters. This suggests that flow at a junction need not seriously disturb the preferred orientation of the red cells, but it is impossible to say whether this behaviour is the exception rather than the rule in the circulation because statistical evidence is not available at present.

The behaviour at converging junctions depends, among other factors, upon the relative sizes of the vessels. In the case of venules of similar diameter it is possible for two streams to come together so smoothly that the plasma layers merge to give a region of reduced concentration in the centre of the collecting vessel which can be followed downstream for many vessel diameters (Stehbens, 1967a) and it has been confirmed that the apparent integrity of the two streams is not an optical artifact by examining fast-frozen sections of the collecting vessel (Wiederhielm et al., 1967). When a small branch joins a main channel, fluorescent photography shows that the side stream often maintains its integrity at the edge of the main stream (Dollery et al., 1967) but information on the precise flow conditions required to produce these phenomena appears to be unavailable and the frequency with which they are observed is uncertain.

When two small vessels (such as capillaries) converge, eddies and flow patterns seem to control the mixing of the two streams and are accompanied by considerable distortion to the cells as they jostle to form a single stream (Brånemark, 1965). A constant flow pattern cannot be expected because the flow rates in the capillary beds are not constant but show a rhythmic intermittency which is caused by vasomotion (Chambers et al., 1946; Barron, 1960). It has been estimated that, at any instant, flow is occurring in only about one-third of the capillaries of a hamster cheek pouch (Berman, 1967) and even when blood is flowing in an individual capillary it may pulsate, but at a considerably lower rate than the heart beat (Harris, 1967; Wayland et al., 1967).

The formed elements in the blood of healthy animals generally do not adhere to each other or to the walls of the vessel. In fact it has been claimed that mutual adherence between cells never occurs in health (Knisely, 1965). On the other hand, slight cell to cell attraction, leading to the formation of rouleaux or aggregates has frequently been reported (Macfarlane, 1961; Bloch, 1963; Schumann *et al.*, 1964) in what could be considered as healthy animals.

Clearance Characteristics

The restrictions on the positions which red cells can assume adjacent to the vessel wall lead to the mean velocity of the red cells exceeding that of the plasma in the microcirculation. The mechanics of this phenomenon are discussed in more detail in Chapter 8 but it follows that the velocity difference should cause the mean concentration of cells in the microcirculation at any instant to be less than in the circulatory system as a whole. This does not always hold (Moffat, 1965) but measurements of the haematocrit in various animal organs which possess extensive microcirculations are given in Table 7.5.

TABLE 7.5

Relative proportions of plasma and red cells in certain organs

Mammal	Tissue or structure	Haematocrit (%)
Dog	Main arteries	43 [1]
Dog	Liver	40 [1]
Dog	Lungs	35 [1]
Dog	Heart	20–25 [1]
Dog	Kidney	15–20 [2]
Dog	Brain, gastrointestinal tract	15–20 [1]
Dog	Spleen	80 [1]
Man	Cranial pool	33–35 [3]

[1] Gibson *et al.* (1946).
[2] Pappenheimer *et al.* (1956).
[3] Oldendorf *et al.* (1965).

The figures must be treated with some reserve because unknown amounts of blood of unknown haematocrit are lost from the tissue samples before determinations are made. The high figure for the spleen can be attributed to its ability to store red cells which are removed from the circulation after infusion and released after haemorrhage (Winton *et al.*, 1962).

A variety of tagging techniques has been used to show that the mean transit time of red cells through various portions of the microcirculation can be some 3–10 per cent less than that of the plasma (Fig. 7.3.) (Dow *et al.*, 1946; Freis *et al.*, 1949; Chinard *et al.*, 1964; Rowlands *et al.*, 1965; Thomas, 1965; Groom, 1967), the difference increasing when the red cells become aggregated (Bergentz *et al.*, 1967b). It has been pointed out (Whitmore, 1960) that this apparent

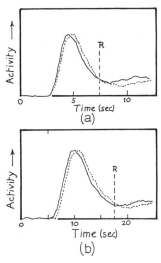

FIG. 7.3. Clearance curves obtained at the carotid artery of the cat of radioactive tracers injected into the innominate vein or the superior vena cava (after Thomas, 1965).

Solid line: ^{32}P-labelled red cells.
Broken line: ^{131}I-labelled albumin (travelling in the plasma).
R: Point at which recirculation commences.

confirmation of the axial accumulation of cells is not completely satisfactory in that in some cases the whole cell curve is displaced in time ahead of the plasma curve (Fig. 7.3b) so that some at least of the cells have apparently succeeded in swimming bodily through the plasma with which they were injected, or the tagged plasma elements have all experienced some delay. It is possible that intermolecular (Philip, 1963; Caro, 1966; Lighthill, 1966) or extravascular diffusion (Goresky, 1963) or even pericapillary flow (Howe *et al.*, 1966) play some part in the mechanism but the most likely explanation lies in the peculiarities of behaviour of two-phase systems in narrow tubes, which are described in Chapter 8.

The Venous System

The primary characteristics of venous flow are that its velocity is less pulsatile (Caro *et al.*, 1961) and, on average, at a lower velocity than in the arterial system (see Tables 7.2 and 7.3). The heart probably does not exert any suction on the blood (Winton *et al.*, 1962; Morkin *et al.*, 1965) but flow is assisted by the contraction of muscles all over the body. Bicuspid, or occasionally tricuspid valves in the veins (Fig. 7.4) help to translate the muscular forces into flow energy by producing an almost immediate resistance to reverse flow after muscle contraction (Alexander, 1963). The rhythmic closing of the inlet valves to the heart causes pressure transients to travel along the pulmonary vein and the venae cavae away from the heart and produces a sharp periodic reduction in flow rate, possibly with some

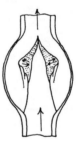

FIG. 7.4. Cross-section of a venous valve, showing the direction of flow of blood (after Clark *et al.*, 1965).

flow reversal (Alexander, 1963; Spencer *et al.*, 1963; Morgan *et al.*, 1966a, b). Changes in pressure in the blood during each cycle are less than one-tenth of those in the arterial system and this is generally attributed to the extreme flexibility of the walls of the veins (see Chapter 2) (Brecher, 1956.) When the pressure inside the walls falls below the pressure in the surrounding tissue the cross-section of the veins becomes ellipsoidal, the ellipticity increasing as the pressure exerted by the blood falls. The flow resistance increases as the tube flattens until the flow presented to the system can be accommodated. A marked rise in pressure only occurs when the cylindrical form is reached and distension commences. Variations in the total blood volume are normally catered for by the degree of dilation or ellipticity at which the veins operate although there is some doubt regarding the proportion of the total blood volume which would normally be held in the venous system (see p. 93). The susceptibility of the veins to changes in their dimensions and cross-section make the reliable measurement of pressure, velocity and volume flow very difficult.

Direct observation of the flow patterns in the venous system is not usually possible but the lower velocities and smaller pulse amplitudes compared with the arteries are usually considered to reduce the possibility of turbulence; simple calculations of tube Reynolds number tend to confirm this (Tables 7.2 and 7.3). They are based, however, on the assumption that the veins are circular in cross-section which is seldom the case; their extreme flexibility permits them to change position with the slightest movement of surrounding tissue and this could well lead to the frequent development of eddies, even if stable turbulence is not achieved (McDonald, 1960b). The valves also act as sources of turbulence and eddy currents in the blood (Clark et al., 1965).

Mean shear rates in the venous system, based on vessels of circular cross-section, are probably sufficiently large to ensure that the non-Newtonian properties of blood are insignificant but the visco-elastic behaviour of the walls of the veins could well be an important factor in determining their dynamic geometry and the energy which they dissipate. Similar experimental and theoretical haemodynamic techniques to those already developed for arterial flow could, no doubt, be employed but the contribution of the rheological properties of the blood and the vessel walls to flow in the venous system still awaits elucidation.

Viscosity Measurements

In order to assess the relative importance of the various blood vessels, organs and circulatory beds to the dissipation of the pressure energy which is provided by the heart it is necessary to measure the pressure and flow velocity in living blood vessels. From a knowledge of their dimensions, or by calibration with a standard fluid, the pressure gradient and the apparent viscosity of the blood can then be found and compared with measurements made in vitro or calculations based on model systems. Such experiments are, however, very difficult to make in practice and give rise to serious instrumentation and physiological problems. In the arteries the flow is pulsating and the pressure gradients are small but various types of flow meters and pressure transducers have been used with considerable success (McDonald, 1960b; Spencer *et al.*, 1963; Attinger, 1964a; Patel *et al.*, 1965; Snell *et al.*, 1965). The microcirculation presents particular problems in that any interference with the arterioles, capillaries or venules is likely to affect significantly the condition of the bed under examination and thus of the parameters which it is desired to measure. Some measurements have been made on flow through the hind limb of a dog (Whittaker *et al.*, 1933), and the long artery of the rat's tail (Kurland *et al.*, 1967), and in both cases the viscosity was found to be appreciably lower than that of the bulk blood after allowance had been made for concentration changes which would be anticipated in vessels of the sizes used. The opportunities for artifacts to creep into such difficult measuring techniques are obvious but the results which are available indicate some of the problems to be faced in the direct application of results from model systems and *in vitro* experiments to living animals.

CHAPTER 8

THEORY OF BLOOD FLOW IN TUBES

A COMPLETE analysis of the behaviour of blood when flowing in a living system cannot be made at present because the full range of variables involved is unknown. But even if this information were available a full understanding would await the discovery of relationships which connected the variables, when a model of the situation could be set up in mathematical terms and predictions made of the influence which a change in one part of the system would have on the whole. At present, attempts are being made to apply simpler models, whose behaviour is already understood, to blood flow under conditions which approximate to those for which the model is true and record the discrepancies between prediction and measurement. As experience grows it should become possible to improve the models until they explain the flow phenomena to the desired degree of accuracy when the complexity of the particular situation may be increased and further refinements made to the models.

The system most amenable to rheological study is the constant, uniform shearing of a large mass of blood and this was examined in Chapter 6. Although it reveals the fundamental flow properties of blood (assuming it to be a homogeneous material) the flow situation is quite different from the vascular system where the blood passes down vessels in which the rate of shear is not constant but falls to zero at the wall and possesses an unknown profile across the vessel. The blood vessel can be represented in its simplest idealized form by a smooth, hard, straight, cylindrical tube and a primary requirement is to find a mathematical model which represents the flow of blood down it. If this could be satisfactorily accomplished, modifications to the model might be made for the presence of bends and junctions, and the flexible, undulating, porous character of the walls. Unfortunately even the simplified situation has defied rigorous analysis but various partial solutions are possible.

Large-diameter Tubes

The flow of a Newtonian fluid down a rigid, straight, hard, cylindrical tube has been exhaustively studied and although there may still be some doubt regarding the exact nature of the turbulence which can develop, mathematical models which predict to a high degree of accuracy the relationship between pressure drop and flow rate are available and were discussed in Chapter 3.

Unsteady Flow

Models representing flow in the aorta and the major arteries of the circulating system must take account of the pulsatile nature of the flow and the distensibility of the vessel. It has been usual to assume that the blood behaves as a Newtonian fluid under these circumstances, and rheological interest has concentrated on the importance of visco-elasticity in the vessel walls. The problem was examined in Chapter 7 and will not be considered further here.

Steady Flow

If the rate of flow of the blood is constant the velocity profile and the relationship between pressure gradient and mean velocity of flow can be obtained for all velocities by assuming that blood obeys the Casson equation [eqn. (1.8)]. The diameter of the vessel should be sufficiently large to ensure that the blood can be treated as a homogeneous fluid and Merrill *et al.* (1965a) established that eqn. (3.16) held satisfactorily for human blood passing down tubes of 130–1000 μ in diameter. They also found that eqn. (3.16) could be approximated to

$$Q_c \frac{\pi R_i^3}{4K_c}\left[\left(\frac{\Delta PR_i}{2l}\right)^{1/2} - \tau_y^{1/2}\right]^2 \qquad (4.10)$$

without serious loss of accuracy.

In contrast, Charm *et al.* (1966) were unable to obtain results for human blood flowing in tubes whose diameters were between 72 and 650 μ which could be explained in terms of a homogeneous fluid and they had to employ a two-fluid shearing-core model (see p. 101) to explain their results. It should also be noted that Charm *et al.* (1962) and Hershey *et al.* (1966) who used tubes of 1–6 mm in diameter treated human blood as a power-law fluid [eqn. (1.4)] and found it necessary to postulate the existence of a region of plasma up to 40 μ in thickness adjacent to the wall in order to explain their results; this may perhaps be accounted for by the poor approximation of blood to a power-law fluid (see p. 65). It will be recalled that different values for the exponent *s* were obtained if viscosity measurements were made in tubes and rotating viscometers. It is therefore not surprising that values for flow resistance obtained in one shearing configuration are inapplicable to another if power-law behaviour is assumed for the blood.

Narrow Tubes

When the diameter of the vessel down which the cells are moving becomes comparable with the diameter of the red cells it is no longer realistic to represent the blood as a homogeneous fluid. Thus in the microcirculation where the cells are of the same order of size as the diameters of arterioles, capillaries and venules a different model must be developed. In particular it must explain the observation that the haematocrit and apparent viscosity of blood fall as the tube diameter is reduced. This is often termed the Fahraeus–Lindqvist effect, after its discoverers (Fahraeus, 1929; Fahraeus *et al.*, 1931). The dual complexity of blood in exhibiting both non-Newtonian flow characteristics and a granular texture makes the problem so difficult that it is at present only possible to consider the influence of the particulate nature of blood on its behaviour in a narrow† or fine‡ tube, assuming in the first place that the cells are rigid (and preferably spherical in shape) and that the suspending fluid is Newtonian. Fortunately the Reynolds numbers are so small in the microcirculation (Tables 7.2, 7.3) that the presence of turbulence is unlikely and any model can be based on viscous flow considerations. Moreover, the density difference between the cells and the plasma is so small that sedimentation effects can probably be ignored under normal conditions of health.

Model Systems

Consider the simple model consisting of a suspension of rigid, equi-sized, non-settling, dispersed spheres suspended in a simple

† A narrow tube is defined as one whose diameter is a number of times larger than the largest linear dimension of the bodies flowing down the tube.
‡ A fine tube is defined as one whose diameter is of the same order of magnitude as the largest linear dimension of the bodies flowing down the tube.

liquid of the same density as the particles flowing at a slow, constant velocity along a straight cylindrical tube. The wall of the tube represents a discontinuity to the particles because they are unable to penetrate it and thus are restricted in the positions which they can take up in the vicinity (Maude *et al.*, 1958; Whitmore, 1960a). No sphere centre can approach nearer to the wall than one sphere radius so that if the cross-section of the tube is divided into narrow concentric annuli, an annulus at the tube wall which is one sphere diameter thick contains a volume concentration of solids which is less than in the main body of the tube (Fig. 8.1). Moreover, the particle–wall interactions in this region are unlikely to be the same in

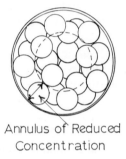

Annulus of Reduced
Concentration

FIG. 8.1. Cross-section of a tube containing a suspension of spheres showing the annulus of reduced concentration within one sphere diameter of the wall.

type or magnitude as the particle–particle interactions occurring in the bulk of the suspension. Thus a reasonable simplification might consist of an axial core of fluid of one viscosity surrounded by an annulus containing liquid of a different viscosity, giving a two-fluid shearing-core type of model. The outer edge of the equivalent liquid annulus must be in contact with the wall and at rest but its exact width need not be specified at this stage so that the spheres (or parts of spheres) which it represents may, or may not, touch the wall.

A number of other models has been devised from time to time to represent the flow of a granular suspension in a tube. Two are of particular importance. In the first the assumption that the shearing, concentric laminae of fluid in the tube are infinitely thin during flow (Fig. 3.5) is replaced by the assumption that there is a finite number of concentric, homogeneous, laminae of equal thickness (Dix *et al.*,

1940) as shown in Fig. 8.2. The rate of shear across each lamina is assumed to be zero while the rate of shear between laminae is infinite. In the case of a suspension of particles whose size is not infinitesimal compared with the tube diameter, the thickness of the laminae could be related to the size of the particles. On this basis the total flow from the tube should not be calculated by an integration of the contributions from an infinite number of co-axial laminae but by a summation of the contributions from a finite number of laminae of finite thickness. This has been termed the "discontinuous" model.

The second, or "wall slip" model, modifies the normal assumption that the tangential velocity of a fluid falls to zero at a wall by assuming that a slip velocity exists at the interface (Perel' man, 1965; Jones,

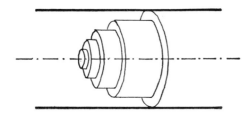

FIG. 8.2. Discontinuous model of the flow of a fluid in a cylindrical tube.

1966; Oka, 1967). This is often presented in terms of a hypothetical layer of the suspending fluid whose thickness is selected to provide the required slip velocity, the main bulk of the suspension behaving as a homogeneous fluid (Schofield *et al.*, 1930; Vand, 1948; Oldroyd, 1949). In practice the thickness of any slip layer is unlikely to exceed about $0 \cdot 1 \mu$ (Silberberg, 1967) and both models are difficult to interpret in physical terms so that only the shearing-core model will be considered in detail.

Concentration Changes. When a suspension of discrete particles flows down a tube it is possible for the volume concentration to be different in the tube from in the feeding or collecting reservoirs. This is because the particles may be displaced radially in the tube by mechanical or hydrodynamic forces, leading to an alteration in their velocity of flow (because of the presence of a velocity profile across the tube) and thus changing their retention time in the tube. In general, if particles are displaced towards the tube axis their velocity rises, the number present in the tube at any instant falls, and thus their volume concentration also falls. Conversely, if particles are displaced towards the tube walls their volume concentration in the tube increases.

Now consider the case of a suspension of uniform spheres of con-centration c_f being fed down a tube of radius R_i. Let it be assumed that they are uniformly distributed in an axial core of radius x, the suspending liquid alone forming the annulus. If the suspension in the core is assumed to shear in a similar fashion to a simple liquid Thomas (1962) has shown theoretically that the mean concentration of spheres in the tube $\bar{c}$ is given by

$$\bar{c} = c_f \left\{ \left(\frac{x}{R_i} \right)^2 + \frac{[1 - (x/R_i)^2]^2}{2[1 - (x/R_i)^2] + (x/R_i)^2 \cdot (1/\eta_{rc})} \right\} \qquad (8.1)$$

where η_{rc} = viscosity of suspension in core, relative to the viscosity of the suspending liquid. Now from continuity considerations

$$\frac{c_c}{\bar{c}} = \left(\frac{R_i}{x} \right)^2 \qquad (8.2)$$

where c_c = volume concentration of spheres in the core. So, if the suspension obeys the equation

$$\eta_r = \frac{1}{1 - K_1 c} \qquad (4.1)$$

$$\frac{1}{\eta_{rc}} = 1 - K_1 c_c = 1 - K_1 \left(\frac{R_i}{x} \right)^2 \bar{c} \qquad (8.3)$$

For a given feed concentration, c_f, the mean concentration in the tube $\bar{c}$ can be found by successive approximation, adjusting the value of x until agreement between eqns. (8.1) and (8.2) is obtained. Also, if the relationship between c and η_{rc} is unknown eqn. (8.3) must be used with an appropriate value for K_1.

Using the experimental results of Maude et al. (1956) for sus-pensions of equi-sized spheres, Thomas found that

$$x = R_i - 0 \cdot 76r$$

where r = radius of a sphere.

Thus the model consists of a core of suspension containing all the spheres and possessing a higher volume concentration than the feed,

surrounded by an annulus of suspending fluid of width equal to
$0.76r$; the mean concentration averaged across the whole tube
cross-section is less than in the feed. However, as we are dealing
with a suspension of discrete particles and not with a continuous
fluid it is necessary to consider carefully the exact nature and position
of the boundary between the core and the annulus. If the core is
assumed to contain the whole of the spheres then the concentration

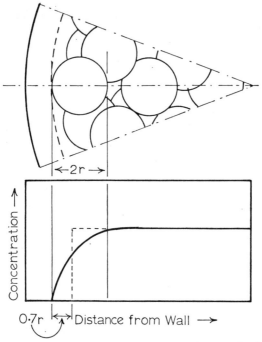

FIG. 8.3. Conditions at the perimeter of a core of spheres flowing down
a tube.

of solids cannot be constant to its outer edge (as required by the
theory) but must fall to zero in successive narrow annuli within one
sphere diameter of the core boundary (Fig. 8.3). From geometrical
considerations it is necessary to slice off the material within about
$0.7r$ of the boundary from the peripheral spheres and redistribute
it between $0.7r$ and $2r$ in order to obtain a uniform concentration
of solids to the edge of the core (Fig. 8.3). In other words,
the outer edges of the spheres would on average protrude about

$0\cdot7r$ into the annulus beyond the outer edge of a hypothetical constant-concentration core. Moreover, the particle interactions which help to raise the viscosity of the core above that of the annulus will be less on the outermost spheres than on those inside the main body. Alternatively, if it is assumed that the presence of each sphere in the core is represented by its centre, the surfaces of the spheres could protrude up a distance r outside the equivalent core of fluid. In either case it may be concluded that the necessity of postulating the presence of an annulus of suspending fluid to explain concentration changes in a suspension flowing down a tube on the basis of a two-fluid shearing-core model cannot be taken as definite evidence of the presence of a continuous layer of fluid at the wall of thickness $0\cdot76r$.

Viscosity Changes. One conclusion which follows from eqn. (8.1) is that the mean concentration of particles in a tube $\bar{c}$ is always less than the concentration in the feed c_f provided that the particles are uniformly distributed across the core. The mean concentration decreases with decreasing tube diameter for a given size of particle so that the apparent viscosity of the suspension also falls as the diameter of the tube is reduced, leading to the Fahraeus–Lindqvist effect. For the two-fluid model considered above it has been shown by various authors (Vand, 1948; Bayliss, 1952; Maude *et al.*, 1958) that

$$\left(\frac{x}{R_i}\right)^4 = \frac{1 - (1/\eta_{ra})}{1 - (1/\eta_{rc})} \tag{8.4}$$

where $\eta_{ra} =$ apparent viscosity, relative to the suspending liquid, as measured in a tube of radius R_i. Using eqns. (8.1) to (8.4) $(x/R_i)^4$ can again be found by successive approximation if the measurements are made in tubes of different diameters and a constant thickness for the annulus is assumed. Thomas (1962) showed that the results of Higginbotham *et al.* (1958) for the viscosities of suspensions of spheres flowing in tubes led to a value of

$$x = R_i - 0\cdot71r.$$

Allowing as before for the core containing particles and not a simple liquid it follows that the thickness of any continuous layer of suspending fluid at the wall must have been extremely small if it was present at all.

Visual observations of suspensions of neutral-density spheres moving along tubes at very low velocities ($Re_t < 10^{-2}$) have failed to establish the presence of a continuous annulus of suspending fluid of measurable thickness at the wall (Karnis *et al.*, 1965). Nevertheless, the existence of some kind of discontinuity at the wall is shown by a difference in velocity between the periphery of a sphere and the wall at the point of near contact, equal to one half of the velocity of the sphere, and attempts have been made to calculate its magnitude (Brenner, 1966). In the wall region particle–particle interactions must disappear and this may help to explain the apparently satisfactory fit of the two-fluid shearing-core model despite the assumption that the core has a smooth outer surface and that particle–wall interactions may be ignored. Measurements by Karnis *et al.* (1965) confirmed that the concentration of sphere centres was uniform across a tube and independent of the velocity flow until $c_f (r/R_i) > 1 \cdot 5$ when the spheres moved almost as a plug near the tube axis. Under shearing conditions spheres exhibited erratic radial displacement but these were reversible so that although the motion of the suspension appeared turbulent it was, in fact, viscous in that all energy losses were through viscous drag and not the result of the exchange of kinetic energy between particles, and the creation of eddies or other random movements in the liquid.

Velocity Effects. As the velocity of flow increases, inertial forces can lead to a radial redistribution of particles. Although a value of Reynolds number of 10 has been mentioned as critical (Sachs *et al.*, 1967), the flow regime is no longer satisfactorily defined by a Reynolds number based solely on tube diameter and a second parameter—the particle Reynolds number Re_p—is required. This has been expressed in various forms (Jeffrey *et al.*, 1965), that used by Goldsmith *et al.* (1967) being given by

$$Re_p = \frac{Re_t}{2} \left(\frac{r}{R_i} \right)^3.$$

If the particle is not of neutral density, various other dimensionless criteria may additionally be required to specify the flow (Saffman, 1965) but as their relative importance is by no means clear and the particle Reynolds number is the most important for systems similar to blood, it alone will be mentioned here.

Inertial effects cause individual, neutral density, rigid spheres flowing down a tube to migrate towards an annulus and this has been termed the Segre–Silberberg effect after its discoverers (Segre *et al.*, 1962). The migration becomes increasingly obvious as the flow rate rises and the tube length increases; Goldsmith *et al.* (1967) reported that the effect was noticeable at particle Reynolds numbers exceeding 10^{-2} although Jeffrey *et al.* (1965) have specified a rather higher value. Segre *et al.* (1962) used a different parameter finding that the effect became marked when

$$\frac{\rho \bar{v} l}{\eta} \left(\frac{r}{R_i} \right)^3 > 0 \cdot 1$$

where l = length of the tube. The sphere-free zone adjacent to the wall is both velocity and concentration dependent (Karnis *et al.*, 1966a). As the concentration rises, the outwardly directed dispersive pressure [eqn. (1.10)] also increases and a subtle balance between the two forces determines the ultimate radial concentration pattern (Whitmore, 1965b). For a given velocity of flow, however, the thickness of the sphere-free zone at the wall falls very rapidly with increasing particle concentration (Whitmore, 1965b; Karnis *et al.*, 1966a) and is barely measurable when concentrations comparable with the haematocrit of normal blood are reached.

Non-spherical Particles. Although at low rates of flow and small concentrations Goldsmith *et al.* (1967) found that rigid discs performed the orbits predicted by Jeffery (1922) at high concentrations they ceased to rotate, their axes of revolution became nearly normal to the direction of flow and their faces were oriented parallel to planes passing through the tube axis (Fig. 8.4) (Goldsmith *et al.*, 1967). At the periphery of the tube a velocity gradient established itself and

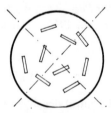

FIG. 8.4. Orientation of high concentrations of discs flowing slowly down a tube.

inhibited-rotations occurred. At high rates of flow individual rigid discs migrated to positions where their faces were oriented in planes passing through the axis of the tube (Fig. 8.5) and exhibited the Segre–Silberberg effect, remaining in an annulus situated approximately half way between the tube axis and the wall.

Flexibility in a particle encourages it to migrate radially, but to the axis of a tube rather than into an annulus. This has been demonstrated for individual rubber discs, flexible rods and liquid droplets (Müller, 1936; Goldsmith *et al.*, 1961).

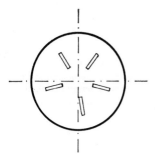

FIG. 8.5. Orientation and equilibrium position of individual discs moving down a tube at high velocities.

Application to Blood

The application to blood of the model discussed above presents a number of difficulties. In the first place the red cells are discoids in their rest position instead of spheres and deform easily. Secondly, the suspending fluid (if it consists of plasma) may exhibit non-Newtonian behaviour. This leads to uncertainty in interpreting changes in the apparent viscosity of blood when measured in narrow tubes in that they can be attributed either to a radial distribution of cells (and thus to a change in their mean concentration) or to the non-Newtonian behaviour of the suspending plasma.

Concentration Changes. Data on the concentration changes in suspensions of red cells flowing in tubes are easier to interpret than viscosity changes but it is remarkable that since the classic work of Fahraeus (1929) and Fahraeus *et al.* (1931) no suitable measurements appear to have been reported. However, Thomas *et al.* (1965) have measured the mean velocity of red cells, v_{cells}, relative to plasma, v_{plasma}, when flowing in narrow tubes. According to Maude *et al.* (1958) these velocities are related to the concentration of red cells in the tube $\bar{c}$, and in the feed c_f by the equation

$$\frac{v_{\text{cells}}}{v_{\text{plasma}}} = \left(\frac{1 - \bar{c}}{\bar{c}}\right)\left(\frac{c_f}{1 - c_f}\right) \tag{8.5}$$

or
$$\frac{\bar{c}}{c_f} = \frac{v_{\text{plasma}}}{v_{\text{cells}}} + \bar{c}\left(1 - \frac{v_{\text{plasma}}}{v_{\text{cells}}}\right). \tag{8.6}$$

The values of $\bar{c}$ and c_f found by Fahraeus et al. (1931) and of $v_{\text{cells}}/v_{\text{plasma}}$ obtained by Thomas et al. (1965) can be used, from eqns. (8.1), (8.2) and (8.6), to find x/R_i (Tables 8.1 and 8.2 respectively) but the problem of specifying exactly the position of the outer

TABLE 8.1

Thickness of peripheral layers
Investigator: Fahraeus et al. (1931)

Feed concentration c_f	Tube radius R_i (μ)	$\dfrac{\bar{c}}{c_f}$	$\dfrac{x}{R_i}$	Thickness of equivalent annulus (μ)	Distance between cells and wall	
					Minimum (μ)	Maximum (μ)
0·405	550	1·00	1·000	0·0	0·0	0·0
0·405	375	0·99	0·995	1·875	0·0	1·675
0·405	225	0·983	0·990	2·25	0·0	2·05
0·405	125	0·968	0·980	2·50	0·2	2·35
0·405	47·5	0·830	0·860	6·65	2·65	6·45
0·405	25	0·692	0·650	8·75	4·75	8·55

TABLE 8.2

Thickness of peripheral layers
Investigator: Thomas et al. (1965)

Feed concentration c_f	Tube radius R_i (μ)	$\dfrac{\bar{c}}{c_f}$	$\dfrac{x}{R_i}$	Thickness of equivalent annulus (μ)	Distance between cells and wall	
					Minimum (μ)	Maximum (μ)
0·38	100	0·952	0·970	3·0	0·0	2·8
0·40	100	0·974	0·985	1·5	0·0	1·3

boundary of the core is even more difficult than in the case of rigid spheres because of the asymmetry and flexibility of the red cells. Two limiting values can be identified. They correspond to cells at the boundary taking up orientations with their faces perpendicular and parallel to the interface. For human cells, an equivalent continuous-liquid core possessing constant volume concentration at all radii (p. 115) could be developed by redistributing material from within about $0 \cdot 2$–$2 \cdot 4 \mu$ of the boundary, depending upon the

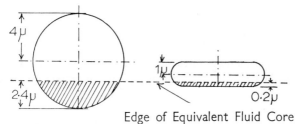

Edge of Equivalent Fluid Core

FIG. 8.6. Limiting orientations of undeformed red cells at the edge of a core of cells.

orientation (Fig. 8.6). In other words, human red cells would protrude on average for a distance of $0 \cdot 2$–$2 \cdot 4 \mu$ from the equivalent core of fluid of radius x. If, alternatively, it is assumed that the presence of each cell is represented by its centre they could protrude up to 4μ from the surface of the equivalent fluid core (Fig. 8.7). The ranges of

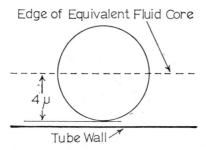

Edge of Equivalent Fluid Core

Tube Wall

FIG. 8.7. Maximum protrusion of a red cell beyond the edge of an equivalent core of fluid.

possible distances between the outer edge of a cell and the wall are then as shown in Tables 8.1 and 8.2. It will be observed that in the case of the results of Thomas *et al.* (1965) (Table 8.2) it is impossible to say with certainty whether cells could be in continuous contact with the walls or not; it would depend upon their orientation at the wall. The results of Fahraeus *et al.* (1931) are also indecisive in the large-bore tubes but acceptance of the theory clearly leads to the conclusion that a wide layer of plasma was present adjacent to the walls of the two narrowest tubes irrespective of the orientation of the cells.

Viscosity Changes. At present viscosity measurements are amenable to analysis in terms of a shearing-core theory only when they have been made at sufficiently high flow rates for non-Newtonian behaviour to be unimportant. This corresponds to a rate of shear at the wall in excess of at least 100 sec^{-1} and preferably 250 sec^{-1} (Chapter 6). Many experimenters have presented insufficient data for a full analysis of their work to be possible and this discussion is restricted to human, bovine and canine cells because they have been most frequently tested.

Haynes *et al.* (1959) suspended human red cells in ACD solution and interpreted their results for flow in tubes varying from 114 to 1494 μ in diameter by means of a simplified form of eqn. (8.1) in which the feed concentration was assumed to equal the core concentration and all terms in x/R_t above the first were ignored (Haynes, 1960). The errors introduced in the thickness of the equivalent annulus by these simplifications are so small in comparison with other unknowns in the experimental technique that they can be ignored. Haynes (1960) found that the thickness of the equivalent annulus of fluid increased considerably with decreasing haematocrit. It was about $2 \cdot 2 \mu$ thick at an haematocrit of 60 per cent so that a clear layer of suspending fluid could have been present adjacent to the wall at all concentrations lower than this and should have amounted to approximately 4 μ at 10 per cent haematocrit. Earlier, Maude *et al.* (1958) had made a comparable analysis of the results of Fahraeus *et al.* (1931) who used human blood in tubes 40–505 μ in diameter, and had found a similar dependence of the width of the equivalent annulus on the haematocrit. They also concluded that the tube diameter was relatively unimportant in determining the width of the equivalent annulus. Charm *et al.* (1966), who used a more complex model in which the core fluid obeyed the Casson equation, also found an equivalent annulus whose mean width was about 2 μ in the case of human blood but it showed considerable variation from experiment to experiment.

Experiments on bovine blood at an haematocrit of 40 per cent in tubes from 58 to 5000 μ in diameter which were made by Kümin (1949) have been re-evaluated by Thomas (1962). The thickness of the equivalent annulus was between $3 \cdot 8$ and 5μ in tubes from 58 to 390μ in diameter, tending to decrease in width with decreasing tube diameter. This broadly confirmed a simplified analysis made by Bayliss (1960) and was in general agreement with the conclusions drawn by Maude *et al.* (1958) on Müller's experiments (1948) on bovine blood in tubes from 76 to $20,000 \mu$ in diameter; they calculated that the thickness of the equivalent annulus at normal haematocrit was about 3μ. The bovine cell is smaller than the human so that in all cases there is the distinct possibility of the existence of a narrow annulus of plasma even if the peripheral cells were oriented with their faces perpendicular to the wall (Fig. 8.7).

Measurements on suspensions of defibrinated canine blood made by Bayliss (1960) in tubes 68 and 960μ in diameter again showed a slight dependence of the thickness of the equivalent annulus on the haematocrit, values of 2μ being obtained at 30 per cent which fell to less than $1 \cdot 2 \mu$ at 53 per cent. Assuming that canine cells are approximately the same size as human (see Table 2.2), the presence of a cell-free layer would again depend upon the orientation of the peripheral cells which was assumed.

On the other hand, Charm *et al.* (1962) used canine blood to calculate the thickness of an equivalent annulus and obtained values which increased from 3 to 40μ in thickness as the tube diameter was increased from 88 to 1082μ. Their model assumed power-law behaviour for the blood and is open to the same criticism as the results of Hershey *et al.* (1966) (see p. 110) but they also observed microscopically that an annulus of plasma 3–5 μ wide was present in the 88μ diameter tube.

Direct observation of flow in tubes is made difficult by refraction in the region adjacent to the wall where a layer of suspending liquid might be expected to develop. From optical density measurements on suspensions of human cells in saline flowing down a tube 190μ in diameter Taylor (1955) deduced the presence of an annulus of suspending liquid at the wall 6–9 μ thick, increasing in thickness with decreasing haematocrit and almost independent of flow rate. The optical density tended to reach a maximum between the tube axis and the wall but this was probably due to cell orientation because sheep cells which exhibited no orientation preference (Taylor *et al.*, 1954) also did not produce the same maximum. Bayliss (1959) re-analysed Taylor's experiments and concluded that there was insufficient reduction in optical density in the peripheral zone for all red cells to have left it. His own experiments in tubes 70–300 μ in diameter on defibrinated canine blood under generally similar conditions to Taylor's failed to disclose a marginal zone but confirmed an increase in optical density at a distance intermediate between the axis of the tube and the wall. Bayliss concluded that if any marginal zone were present it was smaller than could be observed and must be less than 5 μ wide.

Bugliarello et al. (1963, 1965) made measurements on individual human cells suspended in ACD solution when flowing in tubes 40–83 μ in diameter. The concentration of cells fell near the wall but the concept of a cell-free peripheral layer was found to be an idealization, the standard deviation of its thickness being one half to one-third of the layer thickness. Its dimensions were strongly dependent on haematocrit, decreasing from 12 μ at 10 per cent to about 2 μ at 40 per cent but an increase in flow rate gave only a slight increase in mean thickness. At haematocrits exceeding 30 per cent velocity profiles suggested that an off-centre viscosity peak was present, particularly at low flow rates and this was interpreted as a maximum in the red-cell concentration corresponding to the concentration changes found by Segre et al. (1962) for single rigid spheres. The effect was particularly marked in the smallest diameter tube but it is not improbable that additional factors came into play. In contrast, Palmer (1965b), who measured the concentration distribution across a slit of similar width (i.e. 30–35 μ) to the diameters of the tubes used by Bugliarello et al. (1963, 1965) when human blood flowed down it, found a progressive increase in haematocrit from near the wall to the axial plane.

Discussion. It emerges from the various experiments described that no single model is at present capable of explaining the flow behaviour of blood, or suspensions of red cells, in tubes from 40 to 400 μ in diameter. This is to some extent due to the contradictory nature of the experimental data. Most of the work has been restricted to human cells where the importance of haematocrit seems to have been established. At values of less than about 45 per cent direct observation and a shearing-core theory indicate that an appreciable fall in mean concentration of cells occurs near the wall although it is not clear whether the gradient is gradual or abrupt. The mean haematocrit in the tube is decreased (as anticipated from *in vivo* studies, see Table 7.5) leading to a fall in the apparent viscosity. The velocity of flow and the length of the tube have only a minor effect on the distribution of cells compared with the influence of haematocrit (Bayliss, 1952). The relative insensitivity of the thickness of the peripheral layer to changes in flow velocity and tube length suggests that mechanical interactions between the cells and the wall are more important than inertial forces in determining its structure.

As soon as flow commences there would seem to be a marked preference for the red cells to be oriented with their faces parallel to planes passing through the tube axis (particularly at high concentrations) broadly confirming *in vivo* studies (Chapter 7) and paralleling the behaviour of suspensions of rigid discs at low velocities in concentrations above about 30 per cent (Goldsmith *et al.*, 1967). This orientation has a profound influence on the light transmission characteristics of the blood and the interpretation of measurements of relative optical density in terms of haematocrit must be treated with caution for this reason (Kuroda *et al.*, 1963, 1964; Yanami *et al.*, 1964).

The effect of the diameter of the tube on the distribution of cells near the wall is very uncertain. Direct observation and viscosity measurements made *in vitro* on human and bovine blood suggest that if a peripheral zone of suspending fluid is present its thickness is constant or diminishes slightly with decreasing diameter whereas the concentration measurements of Fahraeus *et al.* (1931) indicate the opposite (see Table 8.1). This discrepancy is an important one and awaits further experimental elucidation. In contrast, deductions from viscosity measurements which are not based on a simple shearing-core model give peripheral zones up to $40\,\mu$ in width (Charm *et al.*, 1962; Hershey *et al.*, 1966) and have not been confirmed by direct observation. It must be said, however, that the identification of concentration changes near the wall of a large diameter tube is very difficult to observe except at low haematocrits.

The question of whether the radial distribution of red cells inside the shearing core is constant or not is unresolved. The direct extrapolation of results obtained on model suspensions suggests that cells would tend to migrate to an annulus if they behaved as rigid particles, or to the tube axis if they behaved as liquid droplets. Although in some of the experiments the particle Reynolds numbers were sufficiently large for the migration of single rigid spheres to occur it is unlikely, on the basis of present theories (Goldsmith *et al.*, 1965; Whitmore, 1965b), to have been sufficient to be measurable as a change in viscosity or concentration unless considerable

aggregation of cells into larger units had occurred (Silberberg, 1966).
Palmer (1967a, b) found appreciable migration of aggregates of
cells from the walls of slits 12 μ and 25 μ wide at feed haematocrits
exceeding 30 per cent but solitary cells showed a very much smaller
effect. The shear rate at the wall during these experiments was about
200 sec^{-1} and when the haematocrit was less than 8 per cent regions
completely free of cells developed at the wall. The classic demonstra-
tion by Müller (1936) of the axial accumulation of flexible rubber
discs flowing down a tube is not directly applicable to blood because
of the presence of a scale effect (Whitmore, 1965b).

The velocity profile of the flowing blood is considerably blunted
compared with a Newtonian fluid, particularly at high haematocrits.
At low velocities of flow and in large tubes this can be attributed
to the non-Newtonian behaviour of the bulk blood. In narrow tubes,
however, there is in addition a high velocity gradient at the wall and
the effect of increasing the flow velocity is to make the profile more
nearly parabolic even though the thickness of the peripheral layer
of plasma may increase (Bugliarello et al., 1965).

At normal haematocrits of 40–45 per cent the two-fluid, shearing-
core model in which the outer annulus of fluid possesses a thickness
of one quarter to one half the diameter of a single red cell and a viscosity equal to that of the plasma, while the core has a higher constant viscosity which is directly determined by the concentration of
red cells in it, is probably the best mathematical representation that
has been proposed. It does not necessarily require the presence of a
continuous cell-free zone at the tube wall; this depends upon the
presumed orientation of the peripheral cells, but it is in any case likely
to be very small at normal haematocrits. The equivalent annulus
of plasma can be looked upon as a convenient simplification of the
inevitable fall in concentration of cellular material at a wall which is
determined by complex mechanical and hydrodynamic forces whose
operation is only dimly understood at present.

Nevertheless, there are many indications that at low haematocrits
and moderate rates of flow a layer of suspending fluid develops at the
wall and the thickness of the equivalent annulus increases. This
leads to an appreciable fall in the apparent viscosity of the blood as
measured by its resistance to flow down a tube and could explain
why tube viscometers yield lower intrinsic viscosities for blood than
rotating instruments (see p. 78). As the effect should be velocity
dependent, the apparent viscosity of blood at low haematocrits ought

also to be velocity dependent but this is difficult to detect in the presence of the normal non-Newtonian behaviour of blood.

Most of the experimental work in tubes has been carried out at rates of flow which are similar to those found in the circulating system. The corresponding tube Reynolds numbers based on a single liquid of the same order of viscosity as blood have, therefore, been less than 200 in most cases (Whitmore, 1965b). This corresponds to stable laminar flow for a homogeneous fluid. If the fluid is replaced by a slowly flowing suspension of rigid spheres, a reversal in the direction of flow produces a mirror image of the original flow pattern (Goldsmith *et al.*, 1967) so that although the motions of individual spheres may appear to be irregular, they are in fact governed completely by the streamline flow behaviour of the fluid. Such flow can still be called viscous. It is most unlikely that similar reversibility can be achieved in the case of blood because the cells are very flexible and the relaxation which they undergo following interaction is irreversible but this does not seem to have been tested experimentally. The flow cannot be defined strictly as viscous but neither is it truly turbulent and there is no really satisfactory method of describing the regime.

Fine Tubes

The smallest blood vessels are comparable in diameter to the red cells themselves and the interpretation of flow through them in terms of a shearing-core model is unrealistic. It is necessary to construct a new model if the tubes are less than a few cell diameters wide. This corresponds to conditions in the capillary beds of the microcirculation where observation shows that the cells tend to follow each other axially in single file with their discoidal surfaces roughly perpendicular to the axis of the vessel (Chapter 7). The

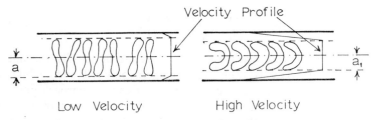

Low Velocity   High Velocity

FIG. 8.8. The axial-train model.

tendency of particles to travel along the centre of a fine tube has been noted by Moreland (1963) and a reasonable model consists of an axial train containing red cells and some suspending fluid, surrounded by an annulus of suspending fluid in which the shearing takes place (Fig. 8.8). The train of cells and interspersed fluid travels as a single cylindrical unit possessing an infinite viscosity. Although it has the virtue of simplicity it makes no allowance for the possibility of secondary, or bolus, flow (p. 132) developing in the gaps between the cells. Substituting the effective radius of a single cell a_1 for the core radius x in eqn. (8.1) and putting

$$\eta_{rc} = \infty$$

$$\bar{c} = \frac{c_f}{2}\left[1 + \left(\frac{a_1}{R_i}\right)^2\right].$$ (8.7)

The concentration of cells in the core c_c then becomes, from eqn. (8.2),

$$c_c = \frac{c_f}{2}\left[1 + \left(\frac{R_i}{a_1}\right)^2\right].$$ (8.8)

This has been termed the axial-train model (Whitmore, 1967b). When the flow is very slow a_1 is equal to the static radius of a blood cell a but it is difficult to assign a particular value when flow increases because the flexibility of the cell and the rate of shear to which it is exposed determine the extent of its deformation. If in a vessel of fixed radius it is assumed that a_1 decreases with increasing flow rate there will be a corresponding rise in concentration of cellular material in the axial train c_c [from eqn. (8.8)] and a fall in the mean tube concentration $\bar{c}$ [from eqn. (8.7) The limiting value of $\bar{c}$ is obtained when the axial train contains no fluid and $c_c = 1$. Substituting this value in eqn. (8.8)

$$\frac{a_1}{R_i} = \sqrt{\left(\frac{c_f}{2 - c_f}\right)}.$$ (8.9)

Once this value is reached a further increase in velocity will not alter $\bar{c}$ because the axial train already contains only cells and no fluid. It is probable that the core concentration does not approach unity unless the feed concentration is high and the tube fairly narrow. In general it is more likely that when $a_1/R_i \simeq 0 \cdot 5$ reorientation and redistribution of the cells commences, leading ultimately to the

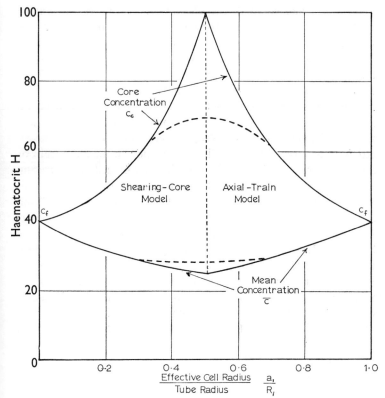

FIG. 8.9. The influence of tube diameter on the concentration of
red cells in a tube, assuming a feed haematocrit of 40 per cent.
Units: Ordinate; per cent.

development of the shearing-core model at smaller values of a_1/R_t.
The presence of an unstable changeover region in which the orientation of the discoidal surfaces of the red cells changes from predominantly normal to the flow (Fig. 8.8) to predominantly parallel
to the flow (Fig. 8.4) might account for the random, tumbling flow
of cells which is sometimes observed in the microcirculation (p. 100).

   Concentration Changes. In Fig. 8.9 the mean cell concentration
and the core concentration in a tube resulting from the axial-train
and shearing-core models are shown for a feed haematocrit of
40 per cent. In the case of the shearing-core model the results of
Rand *et al.* (1964a) at 212 sec^{-1} were used for η_{rc} in conjunction with
eqns. (8.1) and (8.2), and the width of the equivalent annulus

$R_i - x$ was made equal to the effective cell radius a_1. It will be observed from eqn. (8.9) that for a feed haematocrit of 40 per cent the axial-train model can only apply in vessels of less than twice the effective diameter of the cells at which value the core consists entirely of red cells, the mean concentration in the tube then being 25 per cent. As mentioned above, it is improbable that this situation would ever be reached in practice but that a steady transition from an axial train of cells to a shearing core would occur as the vessel diameter was increased or the effective diameter of the cells decreased. Setting an arbitrary limit to cell concentration in the axial train or core at 70 per cent the effect of tube diameter on cell concentration is shown in Fig. 8.9 by a chain line; the mean concentration then falls to a minimum of about 28 per cent. It may be noted that Gibson *et al.* (1946) found haematocrits of less than 20 per cent in some organs which possess an extensive microcirculation (Table 7.5). These abnormally low haematocrits have been explained by the presence of an annular channel surrounding the capillary into which some plasma is filtered and down which it travels at a slower rate than the main mass of blood (Howe *et al.*, 1966) but it is difficult to visualize how such channels could be accommodated in living tissues.

Velocity Effects. Substituting for $\bar{c}$ from eqn. (8.7) in eqn. (8.5) the velocity of the cells v_{cells}, relative to that of the plasma, v_{plasma} in the axial-train region is given by

$$\frac{v_{\text{cells}}}{v_{\text{plasma}}} = \frac{2\left[1 + (a_1/R_i)^2\right]^{-1} - c_f}{1 - c_f}. \tag{8.10}$$

When the cells possess the same radius as the tube $a_1 = R_i$ and the cells and plasma travel at the same velocity. As the tube diameter or the flow velocity increases a_1/R_i falls and the velocity of the cells relative to the plasma rises. It is clear that the velocity difference is a maximum when $\bar{c}$ is a minimum and, from Fig. 8.9, this should be when the diameter of the train is approximately one half of the tube diameter in the case of normal human blood. From eqn. (8.10), taking values of $\bar{c}$ from Fig. 8.9, the mean velocity of the cells would then be about $1 \cdot 6$ to $2 \cdot 0$ times that of the plasma.

One consequence of this result is that if a neutral-density body flows down a tube which fits it fairly closely but does not mechanically impede its movement and the suspending fluid contains neutral-density particles one-fifth to four-fifths of the tube diameter, the mean velocity of the small particles relative to the fluid should be greater than that of the large body. Unless the particles are able to slip past the large body they will concentrate behind it. This has been suggested as a possible mechanism for the hyperconcentration of red cells behind emboli in blood vessels of appropriate diameter (Whitmore, 1966).

Viscosity Changes. Equation (8.4) for the viscosity of a two-fluid system can be applied to the axial-train model by putting the viscosity of the fluid forming the core $\eta_{rc} = \infty$. Then

$$\eta_{ra} = \frac{1}{1 - (a_1/R_i)^4}. \tag{8.11}$$

It is clear that η_{ra} does not depend upon the haematocrit of the feed c_f except in so far as eqn. (8.11) is only applicable if

$$\frac{a_1}{R_i} \geqslant \sqrt{\left(\frac{c_f}{2 - c_f}\right)}.$$

The minimum possible apparent relative viscosity at any feed haematocrit $\eta_{ra(min)}$ is obtained when the axial train contains only cells. From eqns. (8.9) and (8.11) it is given by

$$\eta_{ra\ (min)} = \frac{(2 - c_f)^2}{4\ (1 - c_f)}.$$

At a normal feed haematocrit of 40 per cent this leads to a minimum value of measured viscosity which is only some 7 per cent greater than that of the suspending plasma. It can be compared with an 150 or 200 per cent increase if the measurements are made on bulk blood (Fig. 6.5) and agrees well with the viscosity measurements made on human cells in very fine tubes by Prothero *et al.* (1962a).

In Fig. 8.10 values of η_{ra} are plotted for $a_1/R_i > 0 \cdot 5$ from eqn. (8.11.) For $a_1/R_i < 0 \cdot 5$, η_{ra} has been obtained from eqn. (8.4), assuming a feed haematocrit of 40 per cent, a width for the annulus equal to the effective cell radius and values for η_{rc} obtained earlier for Fig. 8.9. The presence of a minimum measured viscosity in a vessel of a certain size is obvious, the critical diameter being somewhere between 7 and 16 μ for human blood (Whitmore, 1967b). It parallels the report by Dintenfass (1967b) of a minimum viscosity when blood flows down narrow slits and corresponds for shearing-core and axial-train flow to a core containing a minimum of suspending fluid.

When $a_1 = R_i$ the train of cells completely fills the tube and, from eqn. (8.11), $\eta_{ra} = \infty$. The axial-train model is clearly inapplicable under these circumstances but the ease with which single cells can move through capillaries suggests that some lubricating layer is normally present (see p. 102) (Brånemark *et al.*, 1963).

Bolus Flow. The viscous drag of the fluid in the annulus on the fluid in the spaces between the red cells leads to the development of "bolus flow" in the axial-train model (Fig. 8.11), (Prothero *et al.*, 1962a; Goldsmith *et al.*, 1963). The precise conditions required to produce bolus flow are by no means understood but it was shown theoretically by Bugliarello *et al.* (1967) that if the number of boli is decreased by the cells moving in groups the pressure gradient should

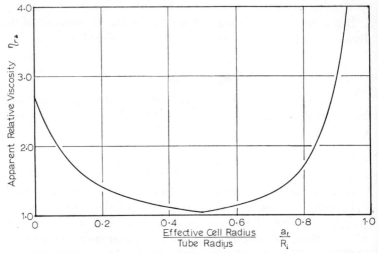

FIG. 8.10. The influence of tube diameter on the apparent viscosity of a suspension of red cells possessing a feed haematocrit of 40 per cent.

also fall. On the other hand, this also minimizes the effectiveness of the exchange process between the plasma and the capillary wall.

Bolus flow might help to explain why the whole of the cell clearance curve is sometimes observed to be displaced relative to the plasma clearance curve (see Fig. 7.3b). An explanatory model is required in which the cells are constrained in a core while plasma exchanges freely between the core and a surrounding plasma annulus (Whitmore, 1960b). This condition is met by bolus flow and it is interesting to note that when blood flowed through tubes of 200 μ diameter, where axial-train flow was not possible, both clearance curves commenced at the same instant (Thomas *et al.*, 1965).

Effective Diameter of Cells. A calculation of the apparent viscosity of blood in very narrow vessels is only possible if the effective diameter of the red cells a_1 is known. The cells distort into various shapes as soon as flow commences, changing their effective diameter (Chapter 7) and this effect is influenced by the flow velocity and the rheological properties of the system. From a simplified model of a deformable body in a narrow tube Charm *et al.* (1967) deduced that the plasma rheology and the elastic modulus of the vessel wall were major influences on the velocity of a single cell, the elastic modulus of the cell being relatively unimportant. The unusual behaviour of red cells in travelling in groups in the microcirculation rather than individually (Monro, 1963) has been attributed by Whitmore (1967b)

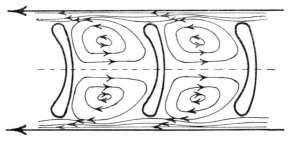

FIG. 8.11. Bolus flow. Streamlines are shown relative to the red cells.

to variations in effective diameter (and possibly flexibility) between individual red cells (see Table 2.4). In a narrow vessel, large or rigid cells will fill a greater proportion of the cross-section than small, flexible cells and, from eqn. (8.10), will attempt to travel slightly slower than the average cells. The small cells will try to travel slightly faster than average cells so that in vessels of certain diameters there should be small groups each headed by a large or rigid cell, or tailed by a small or flexible cell, giving the phenomenon observed by Monro (1963).

It is clear that no single model is at present capable of explaining the flow of blood in straight, cylindrical, hard tubes and the different models which have been suggested for large, narrow and fine tubes must still be considered as speculative. Nevertheless, they do give some indications of possible mechanisms of interaction in flowing blood in the circulating system and are capable of further development.

CHAPTER 9

FLOW IN COMPLEX SITUATIONS

In Chapter 3 the flow in smooth, straight, cylindrical hard-walled tubes of ideal fluids was considered and in Chapter 8 this was extended to include suspensions such as blood. In this chapter the anticipated changes in flow behaviour when the simple tube is replaced by more complex geometrical arrangements which, either singly or in combination, are encountered in the circulating system of living bodies will be examined.

Surface Profile

The influence of the physical character of the inner surface of a tube on the resistance experienced by a fluid passing down it is most marked when the flow is turbulent because the friction coefficient f [eqn. (3.10, p. 44] rises appreciably with the roughness of the surface, increasing the pressure drop down the tube (Prandtl, 1952). If the flow is laminar, the influence of wall roughness is considerably reduced although it can contribute to the establishment of turbulence adjacent to the surface (Levich, 1962).

It is very difficult to ascertain the extent to which the pattern of endothelial cells which lines the inside of a blood vessel (Chapter 2) alters the flow pattern compared with a smooth surface. The importance of surface irregularities normally increases as the velocity of flow over the surface increases; thus in the smallest blood vessels where irregularities in the wall contours, relative to the diameter of the vessel should be greatest, the flow velocity and tube Reynolds number are least. In the largest blood vessels where turbulent flow conditions are approached and wall roughness might significantly alter the flow resistance, the endothelial cells are so small compared with the dimensions of the vessels that the degree of roughness which they represent could be unimportant. Definite evidence does not seem to be available, however, and the general picture is complicated by the suggestion that a biological surface might be the seat of phenomena which markedly change the flow behaviour of a fluid in contact with it (Copley, 1960). The possibility of some proteins denaturing and forming long-chain molecules which attach to the surface and alter the drag characteristics should also not be overlooked (Silberberg, 1967).

Constrictions

It was mentioned in Chapter 7 that the flow of blood to capillary beds is normally controlled by sphincters. The venous valves which assist in the return of blood to the heart also act as constrictions (Clark *et al.*, 1965) although of continuously varying aperture. The cross-sections of some blood vessels may be significantly reduced at certain spots by the formation of plaques on their walls leading ultimately to the complete closure of the vessel by a thrombus in some cases (see Chapter 10).

The total energy of an element of a frictionless, incompressible fluid at any instant is given by the sum of its potential, kinetic and pressure energies; this is *Bernoulli's theorem*. Provided that the velocity (and thus the kinetic energy) of the fluid is large, the assumptions on which Bernoulli's theorem is based are acceptable. If under these circumstances a fluid is moving along a tube arranged so that the potential energy is constant and it passes through a constriction, the increase in velocity will be associated with a decrease in the lateral pressure at the walls along almost the whole length of the constriction (Fig. 9.1). The exception is at the commencement of the contraction region where there will be a small increase in lateral pressure brought about by the redirection of the fluid (Rouse, 1946). Bernoulli effects are only likely to be significant in regions of high flow velocity where the kinetic energy term could be appreciable. This restricts their importance to the arterial, and possibly the venous, systems and the changes in pressure on the walls of blood vessels at constrictions, caused by the Bernoulli phenomenon, are sometimes considered to influence the development of arterial plaques (Texon, 1960; Mitchell *et al.*, 1965). It has also been suggested (Rodbard, 1962) that the growth of the endothelial cells lining the blood vessels is determined by the pressure exerted on them by the blood. If this is true, Rodbard argued that they would develop, proliferate and form cushions in the vicinity of constrictions in a vessel as a consequence of the locally increased velocity and diminished pressure of the blood. One obstacle to the acceptance of the theory is that the slight increase in pressure which occurs upstream of the constriction (see Fig. 9.1) should lead to the discouragement of cell growth in this region. This in turn would increase the inlet taper to the constriction, raising further the pressure in the upstream region and encouraging the elimination of adjacent growth cells. This action would ultimately lead to the cushion being wiped away.

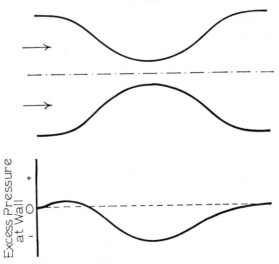

FIG. 9.1. Pressure distribution at the wall of a constriction in a tube.

It was mentioned in Chapter 7 that at some arterial junctions streamlined cushions situated on either side of the branch orifice projected into the lumen of the main trunk and it has been proposed that their function is to modify the haematocrit of the blood flowing into the branch (Fourman *et al.*, 1961). There may also be a reduction in pressure at the intersection because the cushions constitute a constriction, and this might influence the rate of flow of blood down the branch if the flow in the main trunk were fast enough.

A constriction in a blood vessel could play an important part in redistributing red cells in the flowing blood, particularly in cases where the vessel is only a few cell diameters in width. At the inlet, cells situated on the converging streamlines which passed very close to the wall through the constriction should undergo slight radial displacements (Fig. 9.2) (Maude *et al.*, 1958). At the outlet the cells would follow diverging streamlines so that peripheral cells would not necessarily return to their original radial positions although this should ultimately be achieved by the dispersive pressure (see p. 13), aided in some cases by eddying in the fluid. This phenomenon is likely to be of importance only in the microcirculation where the dimensions of the red cells are comparable with the diameters of the blood vessels.

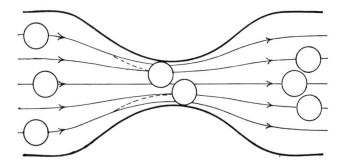

Fig. 9.2. Radial redistribution of suspended bodies after passing through a constriction.

Bends

A characteristic of the circulation is the number and variety of the bends in the blood vessels. In the general case of a fluid in full laminar flow passing round a bend there is an increase in the pressure gradient, accompanied by the phenomenon of secondary flow. The fluid elements which experience the greatest outwardly directed force are those travelling at the highest velocity. Thus elements near the tube axis move outwards and are replaced by slow-flowing fluid from the periphery of the tube. A kind of double vortex appears (Fig. 9.3) which is superimposed on the main flow and causes a spiral type of motion. This, it is claimed, can raise the critical Reynolds number quite appreciably (Goldstein, 1938), and Timm (1942) found that the flow of a simple liquid was laminar in the arch of a model of the human aorta but became turbulent in the straight following section. Entry conditions may have influenced the picture, however, because a single (instead of the anticipated double) vortex developed in the arch. Horlock (1962) discovered that there was no combination of bend-radius/tube-radius ratio and entry conditions which completely restored the original entry flow pattern so that combinations of different bends situated close to each other, such as are common in the circulation, cannot be treated individually. This might explain why Stehbens (1960) observed that turbulence developed in a simple liquid flowing in an S-shaped tube at a Reynolds number of only 550 and could provide a reason for the suggestion by Mitchell *et al.* (1965) that bends in arteries create turbulence. Caro (1966) found the mixing effect to be greatest at bends in model systems where the tube Reynolds number was about 1000. At higher

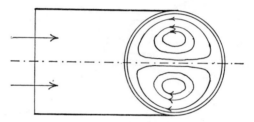

FIG. 9.3. Secondary flow in a bend.

flow rates, upstream instabilities were believed to destroy the parabolic velocity profile and thus reduce the degree of secondary flow in the bend which gave the mixing. The extra pressure gradient attributable to the curvature of a rigid pipe was shown by White (1929) to be immeasurable for simple liquids if

$$Re_t < 40 \sqrt{\left(\frac{R_b}{R_c}\right)}$$

where R_b = mean radius of bend. Figure 9.4 shows the tube Reynolds numbers Re_t at which the extra pressure loss in a bend should become measurable and if read in conjunction with Tables 7.2 and 7.3 leads to the conclusion that if blood can be treated as a simple liquid the influence of curvature on flow resistance in the circulation should only be of importance in the largest vessels. Thomas *et al.* (1963) and Clegg *et al.* (1963) have deduced that the vortex type of velocity profile is virtually unchanged by non-Newtonian flow properties in the fluid and that the presence of an elastic component might even increase the flow rate in a bend but the possible influence of elastic, or visco-elastic, behaviour in the tube walls is unknown.

Experiments by Merrill *et al.* (1965a) on suspensions of human red cells in plasma flowing down plastic tubes 200–900 μ in diameter at tube Reynolds numbers of less than 100 confirmed the insensitivity of the pressure gradient to curvature of the tubes, although the minimum bend-radius/tube-radius ratio used was 10. Song *et al.* (1965) also reached a similar conclusion.

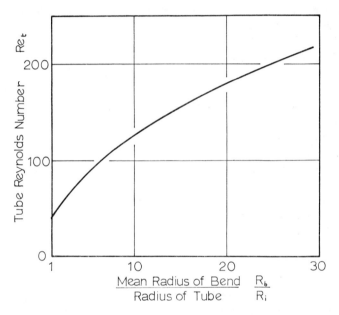

FIG. 9.4. Influence of the radius of a bend on the minimum tube Reynolds number required to produce an increased pressure gradient.

Taper

The only vessels in the circulation which approximate to tubes of constant diameter are capillaries; all others show some taper (Chapter 2). A very slight convergence or divergence in the walls of a tube considerably alters the critical tube Reynolds number and the velocity distribution across the section, leading to a change in the pressure gradient. Only when the Reynolds numbers are very low are divergent and convergent flows completely reversible, and can energy losses associated with velocity changes in the fluid be ignored (Pai, 1956). The problem has been examined theoretically by, for example, Targ (1951), Slezkin (1955), Evans (1962), Oka (1964), Weiss (1964) and Nishimura *et al.* (1965). Experimentally, Prandtl *et al.* (1934) found that convergence tended to stabilize laminar flow, raise the critical tube Reynolds number and flatten the velocity profile, the ratio of the velocity on the tube axis to the mean velocity falling by 5 per cent for a taper of only 20 seconds at a Reynolds number of 2000. In contrast, divergence reduced the critical Reynolds number, decreasing the velocity gradient at the wall and raising it in the middle. Thus there would seem to be more chance of turbulence developing from this source in the venous than in the arterial system for the same velocity of flow in vessels of similar diameter. On the other hand, Attinger (1967) considered that the appreciably greater pressure gradient which he found in large arteries compared with the Poiseuille value might, to some degree, have been due to taper but it is possible that inertial forces made a substantial contribution to the enhanced gradient.

In the microcirculation, the tube Reynolds numbers and the taper angles are so small (see Chapter 2 and Chapter 7) that simplifications in the theories are possible. Song *et al.* (1965) computed the pressure loss by considering the tubes to be composed of incremental straight sections with different diameters, while Merrill *et al.* (1965a) found that the logarithmic mean diameter was the most satisfactory parameter in the physiological range of flow and that there was no detectable difference in pressure gradient for converging and diverging tubes with simple liquids or red cells suspended in plasma. In contrast, Cerny *et al.* (1966), working in a similar range of wall shear stresses, found convergent tubes gave a slightly greater pressure loss than divergent and considered that conditions were particularly favourable there for a radial redistribution of the red cells. Their argument was based on hydrodynamic reasoning but the considerations which should apply to the redistribution of red cells at the outlet to a constriction (see p. 137) should be equally true in the general case of a tube with diverging walls. The angle of taper would normally be very small compared with the flare of a constriction, however, giving a corresponding reduction in the magnitude of the effect.

Cross-section

It was mentioned in Chapter 7 that deviations from circular cross-section are most common in the venous system although some arteries possess a distinctly elliptical section (Attinger, 1964b), especially under normal physiological conditions (Caro et al., 1966). The normal variations in transmural pressure in the venous system are very small compared with those in the arterial system so that the change in the length of the periphery of a vein during flattening is probably very small despite its much thinner walls (Brecher, 1956). It has been suggested that the control of the venous system depends upon this ability to deform (Alexander, 1963).

In laminar flow, considerable variations in the shape of the cross-section of a tube may occur without seriously affecting the discharge (provided that the area is unaltered), an ellipticity of $0 \cdot 875$ diminishing the flow rate by less than 1 per cent (Lamb, 1932). If the tube walls are flexible but not distensible, however, there is an appreciable change in flow rate at low values of ellipticity because the cross-section is drastically reduced. For an elliptical cross-section having sub-axes of b_1 and b_2 the Poiseuille equation (3.5) (p. 42) becomes

$$Q_N = \frac{\Delta P \, \pi \, b_1^3 \, b_2^3}{4l\eta \, (b_1^2 + b_2^2)} \tag{9.1}$$

and the resulting variation in relative flow rate with ellipticity for a perimeter of constant length is shown in Fig. 9.5.

Wall Flexibility

The rheology of the walls of the blood vessels is important for different reasons in different parts of the circulating system. In the arteries the visco-elastic properties influence the transmission of the pressure wave and the energy lost in transporting the blood (see Chapter 7). In the arterioles and the venous system, wall flexibility is used to control the flow rate of the blood although the mechanism is quite different in the two cases (Chapter 7). In the capillaries the whole environment behaves as an elastic gel (Fung et al., 1966) and the elasticity of the walls may have an important influence on the drag experienced by individual red cells (Charm et al., 1967a).

The flow of a real fluid down an elastically walled cylindrical tube distorts its shape into a horn. If the fluid is of very low viscosity,

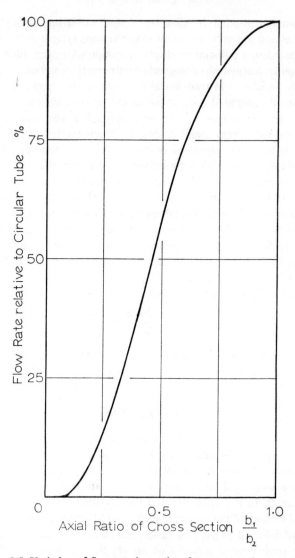

FIG. 9.5. Variation of flow rate in a tube of constant perimeter when the cross-section is deformed into an ellipse. The pressure gradient is assumed to be unchanged.

or the viscous term is small, a straight velocity profile may be assumed across the tube and ordinary horn theory can be used to calculate the pressure gradient (Hall, 1932). When viscous forces are significant, additional terms are introduced and the velocity profile becomes curved but although the general consequences of this have been discussed for the case of arterial flow (Weiss, 1964) no easily usable theory is at present available.

The onset of turbulence is not affected by elasticity in the walls if the flow is steady and the tube is circular (Attinger, 1964b). With an elliptic tube, the elasticity may reduce the critical tube Reynolds number to a value considerably less than 2000 but although these conditions are most likely to be found in the large veins, McDonald (1960) observed that turbulence in the inferior or abdominal vena cava was only in evidence for a very small proportion of each heart beat.

Wall Permeability

The efficient operation of the circulating system ensures that nutrients are transferred to the capillaries of the microcirculation in the quantity and at the time that they are required and that the various waste products are removed from the tissue. These operations require the transfer of fluids across the walls of the capillaries. It is by no means clear, however, to what extent rheology plays a significant part in these operations and they will not be considered further here.

Junctions

The distribution of blood from the aorta to some 10^9 capillaries and its return to the venae cavae is only achieved by passing the blood through a very large number of junctions. In Chapter 2 it was mentioned that the branching patterns are of many different types, the main common feature being that the junctions are normally dichotomous.

The redistribution of a fluid which occurs at any junction leads to changes in the velocity profile in its vicinity and, in some cases, to the development of local turbulence. There may also be a different pressure gradient in a vessel leaving the junction compared with that in an entering vessel and this will depend upon the relative diameters of the vessels and the flow regime. In the case of a simple fluid passing through a junction at which the two branches are of equal diameter, the branch diameter which will give the same pressure gradient as the single tube depends upon the flow regime.

Laminar flow. From eqn. (3.5) (p. 42),

$$\frac{\text{Diameter of branch}}{\text{Diameter of single tube}} = \frac{1}{\sqrt[4]{2}} = 0 \cdot 84.$$

Turbulent flow. From eqn. (3.10), and assuming that f is constant in all tubes (this is unlikely to be exactly true but the simplification makes only a small difference to the result),

$$\frac{\text{Diameter of branch}}{\text{Diameter of single tube}} = \frac{1}{\sqrt[5]{4}} = 0 \cdot 76.$$

Accepted values for the diameter ratio at arterial bifurcations lie between $0 \cdot 80$ (McDonald, 1960) and $0 \cdot 90$ (Caro *et al.*, 1966) so that the question of whether the pressure gradient should be greater in the vessels leaving the junction than in the vessel entering it could depend on the flow regime. Generally speaking, the dimensions of the vessels at arterial and arteriole junctions are such that flow is accompanied by a fall in the tube Reynolds number (see Tables 7.2 and 7.3) and an increase in the stability of flow in the system. The exact geometry of the junction is probably extremely important in determining the flow pattern which develops and experiments have been reported by Attinger (1964b) and Stehbens (1960) to test this effect using simple Newtonian liquids. For side-branching tubes, Knox (1962) found experimentally that the distance of flow of a simple liquid down the branch necessary for steady conditions to re-exert themselves l_1 was given by

$$l_1 = K_4 \, d_i \, Re_t \qquad\qquad (9.2)$$

where K_4 is a constant (varying between $0 \cdot 05$ and $0 \cdot 11$), d_i is the diameter of the branch tube, and Re_t is the tube Reynolds number in the branch.

In Table 9.1 values of the average distance of travel down various blood vessels in different parts of the circulation which would be required in order to re-establish steady flow after a junction are given, on the assumption that K_4 in eqn. (9.2) is equal to $0 \cdot 1$. It is clear that only in the microcirculation is there sufficient distance for streamline flow to re-establish itself quickly and completely after a

TABLE 9.1

Inlet length after branching in canine blood vessels

Vessel	Average length[†] (cm)	Inlet length (cm)	Inlet length / Av. length
Aorta	40	4·4[‡] 167[§]	0·11 4·2
Large arteries	20	3·9	0·02
Terminal arteries	1·0	0·07	0·07
Arterioles	0·2	4×10^{-6}	2×10^{-5}
Capillaries	0·1	$1·6 \times 10^{-7}$	$1·6 \times 10^{-6}$

† From Table 7.2.
‡ Assuming turbulent flow, when $l_i = 1·386 \, R_i Re_t^{1/4}$ (Goldstein, 1938).
§ Assuming maximum Re_t for laminar flow is 2000 and applying eqn. (9.2).

diverging junction. The pulsatile nature of flow in the arterial system serves to aggravate this effect (Atabeck *et al.*, 1964).

At converging junctions having relative dimensions similar to those in the venous system, the tube Reynolds number in the downstream trunk is generally greater than in the feeding limbs and the system is less stable than at a diverging junction. Stehbens (1960) observed turbulence at a Reynolds number of only 200 in a converging T-piece with equal flow rates in the inlet tubes and the same cross-sectional area upstream and downstream. On the other hand, Mc-Donald (1960) found that in a glass model of the Y-junction of the two iliac veins, the secondary flows set up in the approaching bends of the branches (see p. 137) persisted for some distance down the parent trunk (in which the Reynolds number was less than about 1000) but there was no sign of turbulence. At tube Reynolds numbers in the branches and trunks which were considerably below the critical he found vortex rings forming in the junctional region and showing no signs of damping out after travelling 30 tube diameters down the trunk.

If the vessels are long compared with their diameter, the energy losses due to branching may be small in relation to the normal viscous or inertial losses in the vessels and can be neglected. The junctions in the circulation are so frequent that it is unlikely that their influence on the pressure drop throughout the system can be completely neglected, although their effect is probably fairly small in the arterial system (Taylor, 1967) and even less in the veins and microcirculation where the Reynolds numbers are smaller.

Plasma Skimming

The term "plasma skimming" which was first used by Krogh (1922) denotes an unequal distribution of plasma and cells in branching arterioles and capillaries. Although many observers have commented on its occurrence in the microcirculation, quantitative theories and data on model systems using blood or other suspensions are small.

It has already been mentioned in Chapter 8 that the concentration of solids must fall to zero at the wall of a tube so that, when a branch is introduced, the constitution of the mixture discharging from it when flow occurs is unlikely to be the same as in the main tube. Bugliarello *et al.* (1964) found that with a suspension of neutrally buoyant spheres the concentration in a side arm was normally lower than in the main branch and was affected primarily by the ratio of discharges in the two branches, the concentration upstream and the branch size. The concentration in the side arm under suitable conditions may be only a half of that in the main trunk, and if branchings are arranged in series the process can lead rapidly to very low concentrations in some tubes. In the case of blood, Gelin (1961) (using tubes) and Palmer (1965a) (using slits) found that the importance of plasma skimming was greater when the red cells were aggregated into groups than when they were dispersed. Palmer also reported that the haematocrit in a branching slit decreased as the shear rate at the wall of the main slit was raised to about 200 sec^{-1}, above which value there was very little further change, and he attributed this to aggregation at the low flow rates which disappeared as the flow increased. Although the phenomenon of plasma skimming is well known, quantitative data suitable for predicting haematocrit changes in vessels does not seem to be available at present.

Networks

Because the circulating system contains a complex arrangement of branching vessels of different diameters and lengths, the interpretation of its overall behaviour in rheological terms is extremely difficult. Indeed the many attempts which have been made to model part or all of the circulation (for example: Rashevsky, 1960; Warner, 1962; Beneken, 1964; Hill *et al.*, 1964; Noordergraaf *et al.*, 1964; Jager *et al.*, 1965; Taylor, 1966b; Attinger, 1967; Rubinow *et al.*,

1967) have often ignored the peculiar rheological properties of the blood and the vessels because of the difficulty of including them in the model. In the case of the arterial system the assumptions that blood behaves as a simple fluid but the vessels possess visco-elastic properties have led to models which are in reasonable agreement with the experimental data available. The contribution of wall unevenness is probably small enough to ignore in the present state of knowledge, but the roles of constrictions, bends and junctions are uncertain and are generally ignored because of a lack of information regarding the role which they play in the dynamics of the circulation.

The problems are different in the microcirculation. Blood must be treated as a complex two-phase material whose physical properties could be seriously modified in the presence of wall unevenness, constrictions and junctions. On the other hand, wall visco-elasticity is probably of less importance than in the arterial system.

The venous system has been the subject of the least detailed attention and the parameters likely to be of importance from the rheological point of view are therefore the most difficult to identify, although wall visco-elasticity is almost certainly one of them.

At present the comparatively simple networks which have been developed are sufficient to explain many of the gross peculiarities of the circulation. This is not the place for a full discussion of the application of network theory to the circulation but it is clear that as rheological information accumulates on the detailed structure and behaviour of living materials it should become feasible to develop more sophisticated models capable of predicting the performance of the circulation over a wide range of physiological conditions.

CHAPTER 10

RHEOLOGY OF ABNORMALITIES
OF THE CIRCULATION

IT HAS been recognized for many years that changes in the health
or environment of an animal frequently lead to alterations in the
characteristics of the blood and the walls of the circulating vessels.
Indeed the alteration in red-cell stability is the basis of the sedimentation test which is widely used as a quick check on the health of
human patients. Important changes also occur after shock or injury
and following the infusion or injection of a variety of different reagents into the blood stream, including anaesthetics (Barlow *et al.*,
1964). The operating mechanism in each particular case is usually
highly complex and the biochemical reactions involved may be
specific to the particular disorder but one usual result is a modification to the flow properties of the blood. The rheological behaviour
of the walls of the vessels may also be affected in illness, either as a
result of inadequate nutrient exchange brought about by alterations
to the flow characteristics of the blood or through biochemical interactions of various kinds. An examination of all these factors is out
of place in this book but it may be useful to indicate the changes in
the character of blood which are likely to influence its rheology and
to consider how its flow behaviour in the circulation might be affected.
Unfortunately it is very seldom that a single parameter of the blood
alters in shock, illness or disease. Changes in the constitution of the
blood are usually symptoms of a wider malaise which affects other
bodily functions and organs, with inevitable repercussions on the
whole of the system. The resulting balance between the various
influences depends on the intensity and extent of each and will differ
from case to case. Moreover, some of the changes produce subtle
side effects. The fact that, in this chapter, attention is concentrated
on the influence of abnormality on the rheology of blood and blood
vessels does not mean that they are necessarily the only, or even the

148

most important, manifestations of the abnormality. The field is an extremely difficult and complex one and all that can be attempted here is to pick out some of the variables which have either been shown to be important or, from experience in other systems, could be important in the case of living bodies.

The rate of flow of blood in the circulation is influenced primarily by the efficiency of the heart as a pump, the rheology of the blood and the properties of the blood vessels through which it flows. Only the last two of these parameters will be considered here. An impediment in the operation of any part of the system is likely to reduce the efficiency of its nutrient transport and heat transfer functions, and to lead to the development of abnormal pressures in some organs and vessels.

Abnormalities of the Blood

It is convenient to examine first the abnormalities which can be found in each of the constituents of blood and which may be of rheological importance, before looking at the overall picture. Thus abnormalities in plasma and the formed elements will first be considered although in practice a change in one without some change in the other is probably unlikely. Modifications involving the formation of gas bubbles in the blood stream, such as may occur during rapid decompression (Leith, 1966) will be ignored.

Plasma

The viscosity level of normal plasma is determined primarily by the concentration of proteins present. The concentration of lipids in the plasma is so low under normal conditions that changes in viscosity following a rise in the level to unnatural values are virtually immeasurable (Charm et al., 1963). A decrease in the surface tension of dog plasma following large butter-fat meals has, however, been recorded (Swank, 1959) and this could influence the selection of a suitable viscosity-measuring technique for plasmas.

The amount of protein in the circulation reflects a balance between outward filtration at the capillary level and return from the tissue spaces by way of the lymphatic circulation. In other words, the protein concentration in the plasma depends on the balance between the colloid osmotic pressure of the plasma and the dynamics of the circulation. In a healthy adult the concentrations of the various plasma proteins remain surprisingly constant and a vast amount of work has been expended on determining their levels as an aid in diagnosis of disease (Petermann, 1960).

The most frequent quantitative change in the plasma proteins which has been described in conditions of physiological abnormality is a decrease in the albumin concentration (Petermann, 1960) which can fall to half its normal value. It may be caused by decreased synthesis in the liver or loss from the circulation and is paralleled by an inverse correlation between plasma viscosity and albumin concentration (Mayer et al., 1966) indicating that a fall in albumin level is normally accompanied by a rise in the level of other proteins.

An overall glance at the globulins gives the impression that their reaction to disease is a general increase (Petermann, 1960). The α globulins are often elevated following injury or surgery or in the presence of fever or acute infection, while inefficiencies in lipid transport may be reflected by increases in the β globulins. Virtually all types of infection are followed by a rise in γ globulin and in certain diseases (such as myeloma and macroglobulinaemia) new, pathological forms of a globulin-type protein are formed (Putnam, 1960). Elevated fibrinogen levels are usually more transient than elevated globulin levels and marked rises have often been observed after acute injury, when concentrations as great as 0.9 g/100 ml have occasionally been recorded (Gelin, 1965; Wells, 1965). Mayer et al. (1966) found highly significant positive correlations between the plasma viscosity and the concentrations of total protein, fibrinogen and the globulins.

Harkness (1965) has reported that the viscosity of plasma is a useful diagnostic aid. In acute inflammatory conditions the increase in fibrinogen concentration is easily measured as a rise in viscosity. In chronic cases the globulin concentration is also elevated, raising the viscosity still further, the severity of the case being related to the increase in viscosity level. On the other hand, increases in globulin concentration are often accompanied by falls in albumin concentration (Petermann, 1960) so that the interpretation of plasma viscosity in terms of the proportions of different proteins present is difficult and should be treated with caution. Kok (1966), in relating the serum viscosity to diseases involving changes to the globulins, pointed out that the correlation did not allow differentiation between the various disorders.

Infusion fluids (other than natural plasma) are quite likely to alter the viscosity level of plasma when employed *in vivo*. This may be brought about by their possessing unnatural osmotic pressures (initiating transport of body fluids across the capillary walls by diffusion) or by the infusion fluid having a different viscosity from

TABLE 10.1
Viscosity of infusions fluids

Investigator	Fluid	Viscosity (poise)
From Chapter 5	Plasma	0·014–0·016
Gelin *et al.* (1965)	Saline soln. Isotonic	0·010
Groth (1966)	Albumin 10% in isotonic saline	0·017
Groth *et al.* (1964c) } Groth (1966) } Groth *et al.* (1964c)	Dextran 10% in isotonic saline Mol. wt. 40,000 Mol. wt. 1,000,000	0·04–0·05 0·71
Gelin *et al.* (1965) Gelin *et al.* (1965) Gelin *et al.* (1965)	4% in isotonic saline Mol. wt. 40,000 Mol. wt. 80,000 Mol. wt. 800,000	0·016–0·018 0·018–0·020 0·047–0·067

the plasma (see Table 10.1). Isotonic saline and solutions of glucose or albumin (Groth, 1966; Groth *et al.*, 1966) tend to reduce the viscosity level of normal plasma while dextran solutions generally have the reverse effect (Seaman *et al.*, 1965b; Groth, 1966). The viscosity of a dextran solution increases with increasing molecular weight for the same concentration in the infusing solution but it also becomes increasingly hyperosmotic so that the ability of dextran solutions to raise the viscosity level when used *in vivo* may not be as large as the tests carried out *in vitro* suggest (Gelin, 1965; Groth *et al.*, 1966).

The primary result of altering the plasma viscosity is to change the viscosity of the whole blood by the same proportion, provided that the haematocrit is unaltered and no other factors are brought into play. In fact this is seldom the case and it is very usual to find, for example, that the aggregative tendencies of the cells are also altered to some degree. This has a profound effect upon the rheology of the blood particularly at low rates of shear (see Chapter 6), and in many cases is more important than the change in the viscosity level of the plasma. A second factor which must be taken into account when considering whole blood is the change in the haematocrit following an infusion, particularly if an appreciable volume of a hyperosmotic infusion fluid is used (Seaman *et al.*, 1965b; Groth, 1966; Bernstein *et al.*, 1967; Gelin *et al.*, 1967; Wells, 1967).

Formed Elements

Red Cells. In large vessels the flow resistance of blood is determined primarily by its bulk rheological properties. Abnormalities in the size of individual red cells, if unaccompanied by alterations in the haematocrit as a whole, probably have only a minor influence on the general viscosity level because only small differences in the bulk viscosity of blood from animals whose red cells are of appreciably different sizes have been reported (Gregerson *et al.*, 1965). Typical changes in the physical dimensions of cells induced by various diseases are shown in Table 10.2. On the other hand, cell shape is

TABLE 10.2

Dimensions of abnormal human red cells[1]
(Cell sizes from stained film)

	Diameter (μ)	Thickness (μ)	Volume (μ^3)
Normal	7·2	2·0	82
Chronic haemolytic jaundice	6·2	3·0	90
Hypochromic anaemia	6·3	1·7	52
Pernicious anaemia	8·5	2·2	125
Elliptocytosis	7·6–8·7†	5·4–6·3‡	—

[1] Britton (1963).
† Length.
‡ Breadth.

undoubtedly of importance to bulk viscosity; but changes in the geometry of a cell inevitably alter its flexing properties, even if the elastic properties of the membrane and the internal constituents are unaltered, so that the individual importance of shape and flexibility are difficult to separate (Wells, 1964). The experiments of Seaman and Seaman *et al.* (1967) suggest that the major role of cell flexibility is to give non-Newtonian flow properties to blood, while the shape chiefly alters the general level of viscosity (Kuroda *et al.*, 1958). Thus diseases tending to make the cells more compact and spherical (such as elliptocytosis) might be expected to raise the general level of blood viscosity and make it more Newtonian if these were the only changes occurring. The viscosity of a suspension of rigid spheres, relative to the suspending fluid, is about 20 at a concentration of 45 per cent (Rutgers, 1962) so that a five or six fold increase in the viscosity level of normal blood should be possible as the cells approach a spherical shape.

Some changes in cell shape, such as those associated with sickle-cell anaemia (Britton, 1963), severe burns, haemorrhage, nor-adrenaline infusion (Braasch, 1967), high butterfat intake (Swank, 1959) and exposure to hypertonic saline (Ponder, 1948) are accompanied by a transformation of the normal, smooth, outer surface to a crenated form. It is by no means clear how these changes are brought about or what mechanisms are at work in each case but the result should be that suspending fluid will be held in the surface irregularities, increasing the effective volume of the cells and the viscosity of the blood (Ward *et al.*, 1950). Gregerson *et al.* (1967) found that suspensions of crenated cells had a higher viscosity than normal, confirming a report by Dintenfass (1964a) that at high shear rates (where non-Newtonian effects should be minimized) the viscosity of sickle-cell anaemia blood at an haematocrit of 30 per cent rose from about 0·06 poise when oxygenated (and the cells would be of normal shape) to 0·1 poise when deoxygenated (and the cells were sickled). It has also been reported that tissue injury increases the number of cells which have lost the capacity of reversible deformability (Bergentz *et al.*, 1967a) and this again could lead to an increased viscosity level in the blood.

In the narrowest vessels of the microcirculation, changes in the flexibility of the red cells are probably of paramount importance in determining flow resistance. An increase in the size of a cell would be expected to enhance its chances of blocking a narrow vessel unless accompanied by greater flexibility (Braasch, 1967). A tendency towards ellipticity reduces the range of shapes which a cell can assume in the microcirculation at any time while any increase in sphericity probably increases its rigidity, resulting in both cases in an increased resistance to flow.

White Cells and Platelets. In Chapter 6 it was concluded that the normal concentrations of white cells and platelets in the blood are too small for them to influence its rheology directly. Even the tenfold increase in the number of white cells which is possible in cases of severe infection (Britton, 1963) or leukaemia (Bierman, 1961; Britton, 1963) should be insufficient to make a noticeable change in the bulk viscosity of blood. The importance of the white cells, from the flow resistance point of view, lies in their ability to reduce the available open cross-section of blood vessels in the vicinity of an injury by adhering to the walls (see p. 33), and in their role in thrombus formation.

The platelet concentration can also exhibit a tenfold increase, a rise of this magnitude being most probable after severe injury or during certain diseases (Bierman, 1961; Britton, 1963). But, as in the case of white cells, the concentration of platelets under normal conditions is so small that a change in viscosity due to an alteration in platelet concentration should be immeasurable. Nevertheless, platelets play an essential part in the aggregation and clotting of blood (see p. 158 and p. 87 respectively) and it is by these means that they exert an important influence on the resistance to flow. In many cases the activation of white cells and platelets is related to changes in the characteristics of the walls of the blood vessels, which must now be considered.

Blood Vessels

It has already been stressed that changes in the flow properties of blood *in vivo* are generally only a symptom of more fundamental abnormalities in the system. Minor changes in the flow behaviour of blood are compensated, to some extent at least, by the automatic responses of the body which adjust the fluid resistance of the system to give the required rate of flow. In injury or disease, however, important changes in the characteristics of the blood vessels can occur and these may set in motion a series of reactions which ultimately have a profound effect upon the rheology of the blood.

Normal ageing results in an increase in the rigidity of the walls of the blood vessels and a reduction in their flexibility (Roach *et al.*, 1959; Learoyd *et al.*, 1966). The elastic properties of the walls can also be influenced by injury and possibly by diet. Thus Nichol (1955) found a slight increase in the distensibility of dissected arteries from rabbits fed on a fatty diet, but injury to the vessel walls arising from external physical interference, bacterial invasion (McMillan, 1962) or stress (Maggio, 1965) is usually followed by a reduction in their elasticity. Venules are the vessels most susceptible to injury but elongation, increased permeability and tortuosity, localized dilations and finally, rupture of the wall, can occur in most vessels. On the other hand, a high blood pressure is normally accounted for by an abnormal reduction in the radii of arteries and arterioles as a result of stress, obesity, hormones, food intake or heredity (Tuttle et al., 1965; Peterson, 1966).

Protuberances (or plaques) may develop on the vessel walls in vascular diseases. They are apparently particularly liable to form in regions exposed to the full impact of the blood, such as bifurcations, converging boundaries, branches and points of abrupt curvature (McMillan, 1962; Taylor, 1962; Fulton, 1965; Mitchell et al., 1965) so that the possibility of a fluid-mechanics mechanism contributing to their formation has been proposed (Texon, 1960; Rodbard, 1962). Lesions do not become so grossly elevated in the venous system as in the arterial system and they tend to contain very little fat material (Taylor, 1962). They do not appear to disturb the venous circulation in any consistent way but the damage inflicted on the endothelial cells may, in the presence of inflammation, give conditions favourable to thrombus formation in the vessel. In contrast, the protrusion of arterial plaques into the vessel not only reduces the cross-sectional area, leading to an increased flow rate and rate of shear, but may itself initiate platelet activity.

Physiological Factors

Red cells in healthy human or animal subjects are either completely dispersed (Knisely, 1965) or formed into occasional rouleaux (Fahraeus, 1958; Macfarlane, 1961) or loose aggregates (Wells, 1964) which become apparent if the flow velocity is reduced (Schumann et al., 1964) but redisperse when the flow rate returns to normal. The first visual indication of rheological abnormality which is usually observed in the circulation (other than a change in the character of the red cells) is a more conspicuous form of aggregation of the cellular material accompanied by a fall in the flow rate. In some cases it may indicate that the fibrinogen–fibrin reaction (see

Chapter 6) has been activated but the various preliminary steps which are required to promote this reaction are still open to debate, despite intensive research over many years (Biggs *et al.*, 1962). It is fairly clear that one of the most important initiating mechanisms is associated with modifications to the structure of the platelets. These changes, which generally occur after injury to, or interference with, the system can also release agents which are capable of modifying the aggregative tendencies of the red cells.

In the case of direct haemorrhage from a major blood vessel, platelet activity is initially restricted to the area of injury. The activated platelets trigger the fibrinogen–fibrin reaction near the site of the injury but continue to circulate in the system (Swank, 1962; Hissen *et al.*, 1966; Swank *et al.*, 1966b); arterioles contract and slow the flow rate in the microcirculation (Tuttle *et al.*, 1965; Hardaway, 1967; the diffusion of tissue fluids into the circulation through the walls of the capillaries changes the protein balance, and various secretions are released into the system (Gelin, 1961; Maggio, 1965). All these factors contribute in some degree to red-cell aggregation making it difficult to establish the part played by the platelets in the aggregation.

During inflammation which is the almost universal reaction of the living tissues of the higher animals to local damage produced by physical or chemical means (Macfarlane, 1961), the arterioles dilate in the inflamed area and vessels which were previously empty are filled with blood. Leucocytes become sticky and adhere to the walls (Macfarlane, 1961; Merrill *et al.*, 1961; Sanders *et al.*, 1966; Stehbens, 1967b), and the surfaces of red cells passing through the area are given a sticky character (Macfarlane, 1961). Platelet aggregates form on the wall and wash away (Stehbens, 1967a), disperse (Rutty, 1965) or block the small capillaries (Berman, 1967; Fulton *et al.*, 1967), their localized activity encouraging the formation of a fibrin clot behind the platelet aggregate (Berman, 1961). Circulating aggregates of red cells form and block the capillaries (Gelin, 1961; Knisely, 1963) leading to leakage of plasma elements through the wall. This is another fundamental expression of tissue injury (Moon, 1944; Arturson *et al.*, 1961; Arturson *et al.*, 1964) and it increases the local haematocrit (Knisely, 1951). In disease there may additionally be bacterial interference with the red cells, particularly to the surface of the membrane (Bloch *et al.*, 1956), encouraging further their aggregating tendencies.

Thus the usual result of disturbing the balance of the circulating system is to impair its operation and the deterioration may proceed even when the haemorrhage or interference is stopped (Gregerson et al., 1961). The side effects and interactions which follow any particular type of disturbance are many and complex and cannot be considered further here, but from the rheological point of view the important but unresolved question is the extent to which the slowing down of the flow is influenced by contraction of the blood vessels, shape changes or aggregation of the red cells, changes in plasma viscosity, and alterations in the haematocrit. It is interesting to note that during haemorrhage the haematocrit of the whole body falls at much the same rate as the venous haematocrit (Reeve et al., 1953) although there may at the same time be some redistribution of plasma and formed elements between blood vessels of different sizes in the body (Chacalos, 1963; Chacalos et al., 1963).

In the case of vascular disease the course of events leading to interference with the circulating system is rather different and involves a subtle, but still incompletely understood, interplay between the damaged walls and the blood. Whether a plaque on the wall should be looked upon as an injured area on which platelet activity will commence is uncertain but the probability of plaque formation is greater in some parts of the circulation than in others (Mustard et al., 1962; Mitchell et al., 1965). The thrombi consist primarily of amorphous masses of platelet aggregates surrounded by white cells and embedded in a fibrin network (Mitchell et al., 1965; Fulton et al., 1967). In vitro experiments (Rozenberg et al., 1966) showed that the platelet areas in thrombi increased with increasing rate of shear during their formation and it is interesting to note that those formed in the venous system, where flow rates and rates of shear are generally lower than in the arterial system (see Tables 7.2, 7.3 and 7.4) tend to contain fewer platelet masses than arterial thrombi (Paterson, 1962; Rozenberg et al., 1966). The question of whether a predisposition to thrombus formation can be detected from the rheology of the blood is difficult to resolve because measurements are normally only made after a definite impairment to the circulation has been detected, by which time some damage to tissue may have already occurred and initiated the changes in the blood which are associated with it.

Aggregation

The action of aggregation in any suspension, if it is severe enough and the concentration of particles is sufficiently high, is to produce a structure in which each particle constitutes a link in the complete mass. Before the suspension can be sheared, as in a viscometer, the structure must be broken and this reveals itself as a yield stress. It has been shown that the aggregation of dispersed suspensions of particles takes place in stages (Obiakor *et al.*, 1964). A small increase in the attractive inter-particle forces produced individual flocs which sedimented rapidly and gave the suspension only a minute yield stress. A larger increase in the forces led to the immediate formation of a structure which sedimented slowly and gave the suspension a high yield stress. The plastic viscosity also rose with any increase in the strength of the structure and this was attributed to an increase in the effective concentration of the solids, brought about by fluid being held in the interstices of the flocs. The same cycle of events does not appear to apply, however, in the case of blood.

It was pointed out in Chapter 6 that the notable flow characteristics of normal blood are its non-Newtonian behaviour, which becomes significant at rates of shear of less than about 50 sec^{-1}, and the possession of a very small yield stress which is probably attributable to red cell aggregation. The yield stress is usually obtained by extrapolating the shear stress/rate of shear curve of the blood to zero rate of shear (see Chapter 1) but the intercept is quite unreliable unless readings are taken at shear rates well below 1 sec^{-1}. Above this value the non-Newtonian character of normal blood is still obvious but the relative contributions of aggregation and red cell flexibility to this behaviour are unknown. *In vitro* measurements of the viscosity of suspensions of human blood cells, relative to the viscosity of the suspending fluid, show a remarkable constancy at the same haematocrit and rate of shear irrespective of the degree of aggregation present (Gelin *et al.*, 1965; Whitmore, 1967a) (Fig. 10.1). This is true if the suspending fluid is isotonic saline (which maintains the cells in a dispersed state), low molecular-weight dextran (which is believed to inhibit aggregation), normal dextran (which produces slight aggregation) or high molecular-weight dextran (which gives strong aggregation). Even suspensions of red cells of blood group B suspended in normal and pathological A-plasma (which produce strong irreversible aggregation of cells) show similar relative viscosities to B cells suspended in B-plasma. The minimum rate of shear used in these experiments was 21 sec⁻¹ and it must be concluded that at or above this rate of shear, cell aggregation makes an insignificant contribution to flow resistance for the systems described. This is in marked contrast to the behaviour of aggregated suspensions of spheres or clay particles where flow resistance is considerably greater than when the particles are dispersed even at shear rates as high as 500 sec⁻¹ (Obiakor *et al.*, 1964) and it suggests that the type of structure formed by the aggregation of red cells is different from that developed by rigid, non-biological

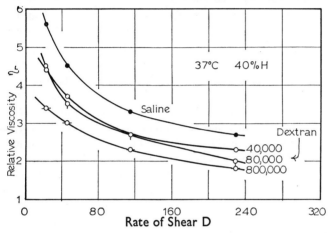

FIG. 10.1. Relative viscosity of suspensions of human red cells in saline and in dextran solutions of different molecular weights.
Units: Abscissa; sec⁻¹.

particles. In particular it points to the cell membranes possessing surface properties which permit some of them to slide over each other with relative ease, even in the presence of strong attractive forces, giving the structure a low yield stress.

The general similarity of the viscosity level of aggregated and dispersed blood at moderate rates of shear should not be taken as proof that the aggregates of red cells have necessarily been dispersed by the shearing action. It is known (Ward *et al.*, 1950) that the bulk viscosity of a suspension of dispersed bodies only becomes dependent upon their size if their surfaces are rough or irregular enough to immobilize some suspending fluid by holding it in the surface indentations and thus increasing the effective volume of each particle.

For a similar reason, fluid immobilized in the interstices of aggregates of rigid particles makes the plastic viscosity of a flocculated suspension greater than the viscosity of the suspension when dispersed. In the case of blood, the flexible nature of the cells probably makes the volume concentration of the aggregates very little different from that of the constituent red cells, so that the viscosity level should be insensitive to aggregation provided that the shape change from biconcave discoids to unspecified aggregates can be ignored. On the other hand, the flexibility of an aggregate is probably much less than that of the individual cells and should make aggregated blood more Newtonian than dispersed blood.

A major difficulty in attempting to relate rheological measurements to red cell aggregation is to define it in quantitative terms. For example, should the degree of aggregation be judged by the size or the form of the aggregates, by the extent to which a complete structure is formed or by the strength of the bonding forces? The answer probably depends upon the part of the living circulation in which the aggregation is occurring. Whether it will impair flow depends upon the size and deformability of the aggregates, their number and location within the circulating system, and their ability to resist the shearing forces of flow that tend to disperse them. Visual evidence is that when aggregation occurs *in vivo* it is most easily detected in the venous system (Wells, 1964, 1965). This is understandable because the slower flow rates (see Tables 7.2 and 7.3) and smaller shear rates (see Table 7.4) prevailing there make the aggregates larger and more easily detected. The mean rates of shear in most of the blood vessels should be high enough under normal circumstances to ensure that aggregation makes an insignificant contribution to the viscosity of the blood. In the smallest vessels, however, or under abnormal physiological conditions which produce severe aggregation, other factors than the bulk viscosity must be taken into consideration.

Occurrence in the Microcirculation

It has been argued (Fahraeus, 1958) that aggregation in the microcirculation might aid blood flow by drawing the cells into a core and increasing the width of the plasma layer in which most of the shear occurs (see Chapter 8). But although experiments have shown (Bergentz *et al.*, 1967b) that the infusion of high-molecular weight dextran in dogs both aggregated the red cells and reduced slightly their transit time (relative to the plasma) when measured between the right atrium and the femoral artery, the absolute transit time of both fractions was considerably increased because the dextran raised the viscosity of the plasma. Thus Fahraeus's argument could not be fully tested but if inter-cell forces were ever large enough to be effective in drawing the cells into a tight core in some vessels the question must be faced of how they would fare when they attempted to reorient themselves at the entrance to, and during flow through, the narrowest vessels. It is difficult to visualize strongly aggregated cells carrying out the necessary re-ordering without creating a large pressure drop and possibly blocking some capillaries (Knisely, 1965). On the other hand, if the aggregative forces were small enough to permit easy reordering of the cells on entering capillaries it is doubtful whether they would be strong enough to influence any axial streaming in larger vessels. On balance it would not be surprising to find that the flow resistance across tissue containing blood vessels of a wide range of diameters increased with the strength of the aggregating bonds if the mean haematocrit and plasma viscosity were held constant. But these conditions would seldom be met in practice because if an appreciable fall in the flow rate were induced, other influences which must now be considered would come into play.

In the first place the vasomotor system might relax the arterioles and increase the number of active capillaries (Maggio, 1965) in order to permit flow to continue. Arteriolo-venular or arterio-venous shunts could open and permit blood to bypass the terminal arterioles which offered high resistance (Chambers et al., 1943; Gelin, 1961). The aggregates could then pass down the vessels if they were present in flexible, distensible masses although their concentration might vary from vessel to vessel. Very severe aggregation, however, is capable of producing much more rigid, compact masses of cells which can distort the walls of the capillaries, ultimately causing complete blockage (Knisely, 1965). If the permeability of the walls increased, albumin would pass through the walls, followed by fibrinogen, globulins and, finally, red cells (Arturson et al., 1961; Arturson, 1964) as the walls became increasingly porous. In such cases the concentration of red cells in the affected capillaries would rise, adding to the flow resistance and ultimately causing some of them to become completely plugged. At the same time the trapping of red cells in the microcirculation would reduce their concentration in the larger vessels which, when combined with the increased settling rate induced by the aggregation, might lead to a settling-out of cells and "gravity layered" flow (Knisely, 1965). If the changes were accompanied by moderate haemorrhage the lost blood would be replaced by formed elements held in the spleen and body fluids diffused through the capillary walls (Gregerson *et al.*, 1961) and although the haematocrit might vary widely from vessel to vessel the mean value could be only marginally altered (Swank, 1962). A broad range of rheological and other properties of the aggregated blood is thus involved and Knisely (1965) has pointed out the difficulty of obtaining a representative sample of blood upon which *in vitro* tests may be made under such conditions.

Aggregating Mechanisms

If a drop of blood from a healthy mammal is brought into contact with glass the red cells often congregate into long chains (or rouleaux) by face to face contact (Macfarlane, 1961), horse cells forming them particularly rapidly *in vitro* although they are normally dispersed *in vivo* (Knisely, 1965). On the other hand, if healthy blood is collected in an anticoagulant, good dispersion of the cells is usually assured for a considerable period of time.

The reason for the onset of aggregation among the red cells in healthy blood is by no means clear and it is most unlikely to be due to a single cause. The biochemistry of the cell and its membrane is complex and has been carefully studied but the rheology which accompanies changes in its aggregative tendencies has received much less attention. The balance of the biological control system which maintains complete or relative dispersion of the cells in normal health is quite delicate and is obviously upset by a variety of factors. It was mentioned in Chapter 2 that red cells normally carry a negative charge and it might be expected that if this were the only force to be considered dispersion of the cells by electrostatic repulsion would always occur so long as it was present. Three main reasons for aggregation can be put forward:

(a) Reduction or complete removal of the surface charge.
(b) Development of adhesive substances on the surfaces of the red cells.
(c) Bridging between cells by certain molecules.

It is unlikely that such a fundamental parameter as the charge on the red cells would change appreciably *in vivo* without some alteration to other characteristics of the blood and possibly to the blood vessels also. These changes could well mask the effect of a different surface charge. Swank *et al.* (1966b) observed a decrease in the mobility of the red cells (corresponding to a fall in surface charge) in dogs after trauma and a change in the blood viscosity which rose by about 20 per cent at a shear rate of $2 \cdot 3$ sec^{-1}, suggesting the development of a yield stress and thus of aggregation. But it was accompanied by a loss in total proteins (which was probably chiefly in the albumin fraction) and this too should have encouraged aggregation. All dextrans of molecular weights between 40,000 and 150,000 cause striking increases in the negative charge on red cells but their aggregating abilities depend upon the molecular weight (Castaneda *et al.*, 1964). Seaman (1967) altered the charge on red cells *in vitro* (including eliminating it completely) without producing a measurable change in the viscosity of a suspension of the cells, but as the measurements were made at rates of shear exceeding about 6 sec^{-1} aggregation, if present, might not have been detectable.

The second mechanism of aggregation is associated with a change in the character of the membrane of the red cells. It develops a sticky protein precipitate (Knisely *et al.*, 1950; Thorsen *et al.*, 1950; Knisely, 1951; Bloch *et al.*, 1956; Macfarlane, 1961) and can produce severe aggregation or "sludging" of the blood, the masses of cells formed being reported to be so rigid in some cases that they distorted the walls of a capillary down which they flowed (Knisely, 1965). Sludging occurs most frequently in infection (Knisely, 1965) after cells have passed through an inflamed vessel (Macfarlane, 1961), and possibly in trauma or allergy (Maggio, 1965).

The third aggregative mechanism involves a direct coupling between red cells by long-chain molecules. Audsley (1965) has shown that such linkages are possible in non-biological systems and the strong aggregating effect on red cells of fibrinogen, some globulins, high molecular-weight dextran, hydroxycellulose and polyvinyl pyrolidine, for example, has been well documented (Thorsen *et al.*, 1950; Cullen *et al.*, 1954; Swank, 1958; Bergentz *et al.*, 1963; Groth *et al.*, 1964a, b, c; Wells *et al.*, 1964; Gelin *et al.*, 1965; Groth *et al.*, 1965; Wells, 1965; Engesett *et al.*, 1966) and was discussed in Chapter 6. There are, however, notable exceptions and some red cells appear to be relatively unaffected by the presence of long-chain molecules (Eliasson *et al.*, 1965). The fibrinogen and globulin levels in the plasma are extremely sensitive to disease or stress (Wells, 1964) and they are probably the main reason for the plasma and serum viscosity being related to the health of a patient (Harkness, 1965; Kok, 1966) but in addition they can have a marked effect on the viscosity of whole blood by aggregating the red cells (see Chapter 6).

The justification for, and the boundaries between, the different mechanisms is by no means clear-cut and it is unresolved whether rouleau formation, aggregation and sludging should be considered as separate phenomena, from the biochemical point of view (which is very probable), or as varying degrees of severity of the same pheno- menon. The marshalling of aggregating red cells into rouleaux requires that the attractive force between the cells should be small and their surfaces smooth so that they can readjust their relative positions after coming into contact in order to present the minimum free surface to the plasma. This corresponds to the rouleau form. It is never seen in suspensions of flocculated spheres or randomly shaped rigid particles but can be demonstrated with cork discs smeared with oil and suspended in water (Norris, 1869). It should be noted that sickle cells (Ponder, 1948; Seaman *et al.*, 1964) and cre- nated cells (Macfarlane, 1961) do not seem capable of forming rouleaux, suggesting that the undulating nature or modified structure of their surfaces inhibits relative movement of the cells after initial contact has been made.

The apparent development of rouleau formations in capillaries may be caused in some cases simply by the necessity for red cells to follow each other in single file down vessels of certain diameters, the groups dispersing at junctions (Monro, 1963). In genuine rouleaux there is a distinct attraction between the cells and a reduction in the mean thickness of each individual member (Burton, 1964).

Clinical Measurements

The viscosity of blood from mammals suffering from a variety of conditions and diseases has been measured on a number of occa- sions. Unfortunately the interpretation of the results as a measure of abnormality is in most cases almost impossible because it is uncertain to what extent plasma viscosity, aggregation, red cell shape and haematocrit have contributed to the overall change. The haematocrit may rise from its normal value of 40 or 45 per cent to as high as 80 per cent if there is a loss of control in the cell-producing mechanism such as occurs in polycythemia. It can also fall to less than 30 per cent by an inhibition of the producer cells outstripping the available supply of new ones (Britton, 1963). In Chapter 6 it was shown that an increase in haematocrit from 30 to 80 per cent gives a three and a half fold increase in viscosity and Rozenberg et al. (1964) found the viscosity of polycythemic blood possessing an haematocrit of 68 per cent to be about double the normal value. It is important to realize, however, that changes in haematocrit are likely to affect the bulk viscosity of blood more than its flow properties in the microcirculation. Most of the shearing in a capillary takes place in the plasma annulus adjacent to the wall (see Chapter 8) and the pressure drop is, therefore, primarily dependent upon the viscous properties of the plasma.

The structure which forms in aggregated blood appears to be remarkably weak and if viscosity measurements are made at shear rates exceeding 2 or 3 sec^{-1} the influence of aggregation is usually quite small. Although very high apparent viscosities have sometimes been recorded at high shear rates after shock (Gelin, 1965; Zederfeldt, 1965) other reports are that the changes are insignificant (Lee, 1966; Swank et al., 1966a) and the evidence is somewhat conflicting in the cases of diabetes and vascular diseases (Pringle et al., 1965; Rosenblatt et al., 1965; Lee, 1966; Skovborg et al., 1966, 1967; Swank et al., 1966a) but with a tendency on the whole towards a raised value. The influence of injections of histamine (Hissen et al., 1966) and thrombin (Groth et al., 1966) in animals which should encourage aggregation has been found to make only a minor difference to the blood viscosity.

When the rate of shear is reduced below about 1 sec^{-1} changes in the circulating blood brought about by vascular diseases (Dintenfass, 1963c, 1967a) multiple myeloma (Wells, 1965) and diabetes (Rees et al., 1967) become significant, presumably because red cell aggregation becomes detectable as an increased yield stress. Evidence from low shear rate viscometry of the presence of aggregation following a raised lipid level is conflicting (Charm et al., 1963; Merrill et al., 1964) and measurements at higher shear rates suggest that the form in which the lipid is present and the particular species of mammal on which the tests are made may influence the result (Swank, 1954, 1956).

It is clear from the data already available that quantitative prediction of changes in the dynamics of blood flow under pathologically abnormal conditions is virtually impossible at present. The system is so complex, the number of interrelated variables so numerous and meaningful measurements so difficult to make that only a few generalizations are possible.

The result of an alteration in the level of the plasma viscosity would seem to be the most predictable in its effect on flow resistance *in vivo*, other factors being unaltered. Changes in the shape or flexibility of the cells and in their concentration might also be related to the rheology of blood in bulk, as measured *in vitro*. The application of this information to living systems presents many difficulties which are probably more easily elucidated in the large blood vessels than in the microcirculation. The most intractable problem is that of aggregation of the formed elements. Not only is this difficult to describe in quantitative terms, but it is also so frequently associated with important changes in the characteristics of the blood vessels and the pathology of the whole system that the application of *in vitro* rheological measurements to the living body must remain highly speculative. In any case the very limited evidence available suggests that the bulk flow properties of heavily aggregated blood, as measured *in vitro* do not correspond to those which control flow in the microcirculation where the influence of aggregation is likely to be greatest. Clearly this is an area in which a good deal more research is required.

CHAPTER 11

CONCLUSIONS

A FULL understanding of the rheology of the circulation is bound to be incomplete at the present time but various general conclusions may be drawn.

The walls of the blood vessels possess complex stress–strain characteristics which normally include some visco-elastic properties. The composite structure of elastin and collagen gives the walls elastic moduli which are strongly dependent upon the stress to which they are exposed, the stiffness increasing rapidly as the stress is raised. The presence of the endothelial cells does not noticeably affect the rheological properties of the walls but in the arterioles the visco-elastic properties of the smooth muscles which constitute a considerable part of the vessel wall must be taken into consideration.

The flow properties of plasma are by no means fully understood and there is considerable doubt regarding the states and conditions under which it behaves as a simple or complex fluid. The ambiguity of the reported results can often be traced to uncertainties in the measuring techniques used but this is not universally true. Any non-Newtonian properties exhibited by plasma are relatively small and it is probably best described as a power-law fluid, the value of the exponent being in general between $0 \cdot 95$ and $1 \cdot 0$.

The rheology of blood is more complex than that of plasma because the system possesses more variables. Mammalian blood at normal haematocrit exhibits an apparent viscosity which falls with increasing rate of shear to an asymptotic value of $0 \cdot 03$ to $0 \cdot 04$ poise. It also possesses a very small yield stress of less than $0 \cdot 1$ dyne/cm^2 and is best described as a Bingham plastic following the Casson equation. The general viscosity level rises with the haematocrit but flow is still possible at values as high as 80 per cent.

If the plasma is replaced by a simple isotonic solution the yield stress disappears but the suspension does not become Newtonian. It exhibits power-law behaviour with an exponent whose value is approximately 0.9. This can be attributed primarily to the flexibility of the red cells although their shape may influence the general viscosity level, particularly at high haematocrits. The serum proteins reduce the power-law exponent of suspensions of cells to about 0·75 (increasing their non-Newtonian character) but the presence of fibrinogen seems essential for the development of a yield stress although its effect is enhanced in some way by the presence of the other plasma constituents. Blood from normal mammals of different species possesses very similar rheological characteristics so far as is known at present and if treated with various reagents which aggregate the red cells its flow properties are often considerably modified. The clotting action which is initiated by tissue injury or the removal of blood from an animal is accompanied by complex changes in its rheology which still await systematic study.

When blood flows in large vessels, such as the main arteries and veins, the flow rate is fast enough for the blood to be treated as a Newtonian fluid although a possible refinement would be to assume Casson-equation behaviour. The visco-elastic properties of the vessels may also have to be taken into account and where this has been done in the arterial system it has led to the conclusion that the energy losses during flow may be due more to the viscosity element in the wall than to that of the blood.

In the smaller blood vessels it no longer becomes realistic to look on blood as a homogeneous fluid and its two-phase character causes the haematocrit and the viscosity level to fall until a minimum value is obtained in vessels of the order of 7–16 μ in diameter in the case of human blood. The rheological properties of the individual red cells probably become extremely important in determining flow resistance in these vessels but it is uncertain whether and to what extent the walls play an important part in regulating the resistance.

The influence of the geometry of the blood vessels on flow resistance and behaviour depends upon the size of the vessel under consideration. Thus bends are more likely to alter the resistance and flow pattern of large vessels than small whereas junctions should induce haematocrit changes in the small vessels by plasma skimming but increase flow resistance in the large vessels by causing turbulence.

Important changes in the flow behaviour of blood follow aggregation of the red cells when induced by the infusion or addition of suitable reagents or by abnormal pathological conditions, although the aggregating mechanism is not necessarily the same in each case.

It reduces the stability and increases the yield stress of bulk blood, while in small vessels it may initiate an important series of reactions terminating in the blocking of the vessels and damage to the tissue.

Most of these conclusions are still tentative and await unequivocal confirmation. However, the general relevance of rheology to the circulation has certainly been established and many of the important parameters have been identified.

REFERENCES

ALEXANDER, R. S. (1963) The peripheral venous system, *Handbook of Physiology*, Sect. 2. Circulation, ed. Hamilton, W. F. and Dow, P., Am. Physiol. Soc., Washington, pp. 1075–98.

APTER, J. T. (1964) Mathematical development of a physical model of some visco-elastic properties of the aorta, *Bull. math. Biophys.* **26**, 367–87.

APTER, J. T., RABINOWITZ, M. and CUMMINGS, D. H. (1966) Correlation of visco-elastic properties of large arteries with microscopic structure, *Circulation Res.* **19**, 104–21.

ARTURSON, G. (1964) The changes in capillary filtration, diffusion and permeability in experimental burns, *Bibl. anat.* **7**, 453–9.

ARTURSON, G. and WALLENIUS, G. (1961) The molecular "sieving" of the capillary membrane after thermal trauma, *Bibl. anat.* **1**, 66–72.

ATABECK, H. B., CHANG, C. C. and FINGERSON, L. M. (1964) Measurement of laminar oscillatory flow in the inlet end of a circular tube, *Physics Med. Biol.* **9**, 219–27.

ATTINGER, E. O. (1963) Pressure transmission in pulmonary arteries related to frequency and geometry, *Circulation Res.* **12**, 623–41.

ATTINGER, E. O. (1964a) The cardiovascular system, *Pulsatile Blood Flow*, ed. Attinger, E. O., McGraw-Hill, New York, pp. 1–14.

ATTINGER, E. O. (1964b) Flow patterns and vascular geometry, *Pulsatile Blood Flow*, ed. Attinger, E. O., McGraw-Hill, New York, pp. 179–98.

ATTINGER, E. O. (1967) Modelling of pressure-flow relations in arteries and veins, (Abstract) *Biorheol.* **4**, 84.

ATTINGER, E. O., SUGAWARA, H., NAVARRO, A., RICCETTO, A. and MARTIN, R. (1966) Pressure-flow relations in dog arteries, *Circulation Res.* **19**, 230–46.

AUDSLEY, A. and FURSEY, A. (1965) Examination of a polysaccharide flocculant and flocculated kaolinite by electron microscopy, *Nature (London)* **208**, 753–4.

AZUMA, T. (1964) The flow of blood through blood vessels, *Biorheol.* **2**, 159–60.

BAGNOLD, R. A. (1954) Experiments on a gravity free dispersion of large solid spheres in a Newtonian fluid under shear, *Proc. Roy. Soc. A*, **225**, 49–63.

BARLOW, G. and KNOTT, D. H. (1964) Hemodynamic alterations after 30 minutes of pentobarbital sodium anesthesia in dogs, *Am. J. Physiol.* **207**, 764–6.

BARR, G. (1931) *A Monograph of Viscometry*, University Press, Oxford.

BARRON, D. H. (1960) Vasomotor regulation, *Medical Physiology and Biophysics*, 18th edn., ed. Ruch, T. C. and Fulton, J. W., Saunders, Philadelphia, pp. 691–707.

BATEMAN, J. B., HSU, S. S., KNUDSEN, J. P. and YUDOWITCH, K. L. (1953) Hemoglobin spacing in erythrocytes, *Archs. Biochem. Biophys.* **45**, 411–22.

BAYLISS, L. E. (1952) Rheology of blood and lymph, *Deformation and Flow in Biological Systems*, ed. Frey-Wyssling, A., North Holland, Amsterdam, pp. 355–418.

BAYLISS, L. E. (1959) The axial drift of the red cells when blood flows in narrow tubes, *J. Physiol.* **149**, 593–613.

BAYLISS, L. E. (1960) The anomalous viscosity of blood, *Flow Properties of Blood*, ed. Copley, A. L. and Stainsby, G., Pergamon, London, pp. 29–59.

BELL, G. H., DAVIDSON, J. N. and Scaborough, H. (1961) *Textbook of Physiology and Biochemistry*, 5th edn., Livingstone, Edinburgh.

BENEKEN, J. E. W. (1964) Electronic analog computer model of the human blood circulation, *Pulsatile Blood Flow*, ed. Attinger, E. O., McGraw-Hill, New York, pp. 423–32.

BERGEL, D. H. (1961a) The static elastic properties of the arterial wall, *J. Physiol.* **156**, 445–57.

BERGEL, D. H. (1961b) The dynamic elastic properties of the arterial wall, *J. Physiol.* **156**, 458–69.

BERGEL, D. H. (1964) Arterial viscoelasticity, *Pulsatile Blood Flow*, ed. Attinger, E. O., McGraw-Hill, New York, pp. 275–90.

BERGEL, D. H. (1966) Stress–strain properties of blood vessels, *Lab. Pract.* **15**, 77–81.

BERGENTZ, S. E., FAJERS, C. M., GELIN, L. E. and RUDENSTAM, C. M. (1963) Intravascular aggregation of long duration and its consequences, *Israel J. exp. Med.* **11**, 123.

BERGENTZ, S. E. and DANON, E. (1967a) The effect of remote trauma on the red cell, *Bibl. anat.* **9**, 104–11.

BERGENTZ, S. E., LEANDOER, L. and LEWIS, D. H. (1967b) Induced red cell aggregation and the transit time of red cells and plasma through the lung, *Bibl. anat.* **9**, 304–10.

BERMAN, H. (1961) Pathology of the microcirculation, *Blood Vessels and Lymphatics*, ed. Abramson, D. I., Academic Press, New York, pp. 170–91.

BERMAN, H. (1964) Rheological properties of the microvasculature, *Bibl. anat.* **7**, 29–34.

BERMAN, H. (1967) Suppression of *in vivo* injury—induced platelet thrombosis by inhibitors of adenosine diphosphate thrombotic activity. *Bibl. anat.* **2**, 92–7.

BERNSTEIN, E. F. and EVANS, R. L. (1960) Low molecular weight dextran, *J. Am. med. Ass.* **174**, 1417–22.

BERNSTEIN, E. F. and CASTANEDA, A. R. (1967) The importance of low shear rate blood viscometry in extracorporeal circulation. (Abstract) *Biorheol.* **4**, 89–90.

BIERMAN, H. R. (1961) Homeostasis of the blood cell elements, *Functions of the Blood*, ed. Macfarlane, R. G. and Robb-Smith, A. H. T., Academic Press, London, pp. 350–418.

BIGGS, R. and MACFARLANE, R. G. (1962) *Human Blood Coagulation and its Disorders*, Blackwell, Oxford.

BINGHAM, E. C. and ROEPKE, R. R. (1944) The rheology of blood III, *J. gen. Physiol.* **28**, 79–93.

BISHOP, C. (1964) Overall red cell metabolism, *The Red Blood Cell*, ed. Bishop, C. and Surgenor, D. M., Academic Press, New York, pp. 147–88.

BLOCH, E. H. (1962) A quantitative study of the hemodynamics in the living microvascular system, *Am. J. Anat.* **110**, 125–54.

BLOCH, E. H. (1963) Rheology and the dynamic anatomy of the microvascular system, *Trans. Soc. Rheol.* **7**, 9–18.

BLOCH, E. H. (1966a) Analysis of blood flow with high speed cine-photography, *Proc. Fourth Europ. Conf. on Microcirc., Cambridge*, Abstract F.1.

BLOCH, E. H. (1966b) Principles of the microvascular system, *Investigative Ophthalmology* **5**, 250–5.

BLOCH, E. H., POWELL. A., MERYMAN, H. T., WARNER L. and KAFIG, E. (1956) A comparison of the surfaces of human erythrocytes from health and disease by *in vivo* light microscopy and *in vitro* electron microscopy, *Angiology* **7**, 479–94.

BOARDMAN, G. and WHITMORE, R. L. (1961) The static measurement of yield stress, *Lab. Pract.* **10**, 782–5.

BOARDMAN, G. and WHITMORE, R. L. (1963) The behaviour of a Bingham fluid in the cone-and-plate viscometer, *Br. J. appl. Phys.* **14**, 391–5.

BOGUE, D. C. and METZNER, A. B. (1963) Velocity profiles in turbulent pipe flow, *Ind. Engng. Chem.-Fundls.* **2**, 143–9.

BRAASCH, D. (1967) Erythrocyte flexibility and blood flow resistance in capillaries with a diameter of less than 20 microns. *Bibl. anat.* **9**, 272–5.

BRÅNEMARK, P. I. (1965) Intracapillary rheological phenomena, *Proc. Fourth Int. Congr. on Rheol. 4, Symp. on Biorheol.*, ed. Copley, A. L., Interscience, New York, pp. 459–73.

BRÅNEMARK, P. I., and LINDSTRÖM, J. (1963) Shape of circulating blood corpuscles, *Biorheol.* **1**, 139–43.

BRECHER, G. A. (1956) *Venous Return*, Grune & Stratton, New York.

BRENNER, H. (1966) Quoted by Karnis *et al.* (1966b).

BRITTON, C. J. C. (1963) *Disorders of the Blood*, 9th edn., Churchill, London.

BRUNDAGE, J. T. (1934) Blood and plasma viscosity determined by the method of concentric cylinders, *Am. J. Physiol.* **110**, 659–65.

BUCK, R. C. (1963) Histogenesis and morphology of arterial tissue, *Atherosclerosis and its Origin*, ed. Sandler, M. and Bourne, G. H., Academic Press, New York, pp. 1–38.

BUGLIARELLO, G. and HAYDEN, J. W. (1963) Detailed characteristics of the flow of blood *in vitro*, *Trans. Soc. Rheol.* **7**, 209–30.

BUGLIARELLO, G. and HSIAO, G. C. C. (1964) Phase separation of suspensions flowing through bifurcations, *Science* **143**, 469–71.

BUGLIARELLO, G., KAPUR, C. and HSIAO, G. (1965) The profile viscosity and other characteristics of blood flow in a non-uniform shear field, *Proc. Fourth Int. Congr. on Rheol. 4, Symp. on Biorheol.*, ed. Copley, A. L., Interscience, New York, pp. 351–70.

BUGLIARELLO, G., DAY, H. J., BRANDT, A., EGGENBERGER, E. J. and HSIAO, G. C. C. (1967) Model studies of the hydrodynamic characteristics of an erythrocyte. (Abstract). *Biorheol.*, **4**, 85.

BURGMAN, J. O., FORSLIND, E., GROTH, C. G. and THORSEN, G. (1964) Structural rheology properties of blood plasma, *Bibl. anat.* **7**, 399–403.

BURTON, A. C. (1954) Relation of structure to function of the tissues of the wall of blood vessels, *Physiol. Rev.* **34**, 619–42.

BURTON, A. C. (1962) Physical principles of circulatory phenomena, *Handbook of Physiology*, Sect. 2, Circulation, ed. Hamilton, W. F. and Dow, P., Am. Physiol. Soc., Washington, pp. 85–106.

BURTON, A. C. (1964) Private communication.

BURTON, A. C. (1965) *Physiology and Biophysics of the Circulation*, Year Book Med., Chicago.

CARO, C. G. (1966) The dispersion of indicator flowing through simplified models of the circulation and its relevance to velocity profile in blood vessels, *J. Physiol.* **185**, 501–19.

CARO, C. G. and MCDONALD, D. A. (1961) The relation of pulsatile pressure and flow in the pulmonary vascular bed, *J. Physiol.* **157**, 426–53.

CARO, C. G. and SAFFMAN, P. G. (1966) Extensibility of blood vessels in isolated rabbit lungs, *J. Physiol.* **178**, 193–210.

CARTON, R. W., DAINAUSKAS, J. and CLARK, J. W. (1962) Elastic properties of single elastic fibres, *J. appl. Physiol.* **17**, 547–51.

CASSON, N. (1959) A flow equation for pigment-oil suspensions of the printing ink type, *Rheology of Disperse systems*, ed. Mill, C. C., Pergamon, London, pp. 84–102.

174   REFERENCES

CASTANEDA, A. R., BERNSTEIN, E., BANGSTADT, F. and VARCO, R. L. (1964) The effect of polyvinylpyrrolidone, mannitol, dextrose and various dextrans on red blood cell charge, *Bibl. anat.* 7, 262–6.

CERNY, L. C. (1963) A region of Newtonian flow for whole blood, *Biorheol.* 1, 159–65.

CERNY, L. C., COOK, F. B. and WALKER, C. C. (1962) Rheology of blood, *Am. J. Physiol.* 202, 1188–94.

CERNY, L. C. and WALAWENDER, W. P. (1966) Blood flow in rigid tapered tubes, *Am. J. Physiol.* 210, 341–6.

CHACALOS, E. H. (1963) Induced changes in the small vessel volume as determined by rheological relationships, *Am. J. Physiol.* 205, 518–26.

CHACALOS, E. H. and MOORE, J. C. (1963) Effect of the spleen in norepinephrine action on blood volumes of the dog, *Am. J. Physiol.* 205, 511–17.

CHAMBERS, R., ZWEIFACH, B. W. and LOWENSTEIN, B. E. (1943) Circulatory reactions of rats traumatized in the Noble-Collip drum, *Am. J. Physiol.* 139, 123–8.

CHAMBERS, R. and ZWEIFACH, B. W. (1946) Functional activity of the blood capillary bed, with special reference to visceral tissue, *Ann. N.Y. Acad. Sci.* 46, 683–95.

CHARM, S. and KURLAND, G. S. (1962) Tube flow behaviour and shear stress/shear rate characteristics of canine blood, *Am. J. Physiol.* 203, 417–21.

CHARM, S., McCOMIS, W., TEJADA, C. and KURLAND, G. (1963) Effect of a fatty meal on whole blood and plasma viscosity, *J. appl. Physiol.* 18, 1217–20.

CHARM, S. and KURLAND, G. S. (1965) Viscometry of human blood for shear rates of 0–100,000 sec⁻¹, *Nature (London)* 206, 617–18.

CHARM, S., KURLAND, G. S. and BROWN, S. L. (1966) The flow characteristics of blood suspensions, *Biomedical Fluid Mech. Symp.*, *Colorado*, Am. Soc. Mech. Engrs., pp. 89–93.

CHARM, S. E. and NELSON, F. (1967) Red cell deformation and flow in capillaries, *Bibl. anat.* 9, 246–51.

CHIEN, S., USAMI, S., TAYLOR, H. M., LUNDBERG, J. L. and GREGERSON, M. I. (1966) Effects of hematocrit and plasma proteins on human blood rheology at low shear rates, *J. appl. Physiol.* 21, 81–7.

CHINARD, F. P., ENNS, T. and NOLAN, M. F. (1964) Arterial hematocrit and separation of cells and plasma in the dog kidney, *Am. J. Physiol.* 207, 128–32.

CLARK, C., COTTON, L. T. and ZAREK, J. M. (1965) Venous blood flow characteristics, *Biomechanics and Related Bio-engineering Topics*, ed. Kenedi, R. M., Pergamon, London, pp. 265–84.

CLEGG, D. B. and POWER, G. (1963) Flow of a Bingham fluid in a slightly curved tube, *Appl. scient. Res.* A 12, 199–212.

COKELET, G. R., MERRILL, E. W., GILLILAND, E. R., SHIN, H., BRITTEN, A. and WELLS, R. E. (1963) The rheology of human blood—measurement near and at zero rate of shear, *Trans. Soc. Rheol.* 7, 303–17.

COPLEY, A. L. (1960) Apparent viscosity and wall adherence of blood systems, *Flow Properties of Blood*, ed. Copley, A. L. and Stainsby, G., Pergamon, London, pp. 97–117.

COPLEY, A. L., KRCHMA, L. C. and WHITNEY, M. E. (1942) Viscosity studies and anomalous flow properties of human blood systems with heparin and other anticoagulants, *J. gen. Physiol.* 26, 49–64.

COPLEY, A. L. and SCOTT BLAIR, G. W. (1960) Haemorheological method for the study of blood systems and of processes in blood coagulation, *Flow Properties of Blood*, ed. Copley, A. L. and Stainsby, G., Pergamon, London, pp. 412–7.

COPLEY, A. L. and STAPLE, P. H. (1962) Haemorheological studies on the plasmatic zone in the microcirculation of the cheek pouch of Chinese and Syrian hamsters, *Biorheol.* **1**, 3–14.

COPLEY, A. L., GLOVER, F. A. and SCOTT BLAIR, G. W. (1964) The wettability of fibrinised surfaces and of living vascular endothelium by blood, *Biorheol.* **2**, 29–35.

COPLEY, A. L., LUCHINI, B. W. and WHELAN, E. W. (1967) On the role of fibrinogen–fibrin complexes in erythrocyte aggregation and flow properties of blood. (Abstract). *Biorheol.* **4**, 87.

CRIDDLE, D. W. (1960) The viscosity and elasticity of interfaces, *Rheology*, vol. 3, ed. Eirich, F. R., Academic Press, New York, pp. 429–42.

CULLEN, C. F. and SWANK, R. L. (1954) Intravascular aggregation and adhesiveness of the blood elements associated with alimentary lipemia and injections of large molecular substances, *Circulation* **9**, 335–46.

DACIE, J. V. (1956) *Practical Haematology*, 2nd edn., Churchill, London.

DANIELLI, J. F. (1958) Surface chemistry and cell membranes, *Surface Phenomena in Chemistry and Biology*, ed. Danielli, J. F. and Riddiford, A. C., Pergamon, London, pp. 246–65.

DANON, D. (1967) Reversible deformability and mechanical fragility as a function of red cell age. (Abstract), *Biorheol.* **4**, 92

DARMADY, E. M. and DAVENPORT, S. G. T. (1963) *Haematological Technique*, Churchill, London.

DAUGHERTY, R. L. and FRANZINI, J. B. (1965) *Fluid Mechanics with Engineering Applications*, McGraw-Hill, New York.

DAVSON, H. and EGGLETON, M. G. (1962) *Principles of Human Physiology*, 13th edn., Churchill, London.

DINSDALE, A. and MOORE, F. (1962) *Viscosity and its Measurement*, Chapman & Hall, London.

DINTENFASS, L. (1962) Consideration of the internal viscosity of red cells and its effect on the viscosity of whole blood, *Angiology* **13**, 333–44.

DINTENFASS, L. (1963a) A study in flow, viscosity and clotting of human blood, *Med. J. Aust.* **1**, 575–8.

DINTENFASS, L. (1963b) An application of a cone-in-cone viscometer to the study of viscosity, thixotropy and clotting of whole blood, *Biorheol.* **1**, 91–9.

DINTENFASS, L. (1963c) Blood rheology in cardio-vascular diseases, *Nature (London)*, **199**, 813–15.

DINTENFASS, L. (1964a) Molecular and rheological considerations of the red cell membrane in view of the internal fluidity of the red cell, *Acta haemat.* **32**, 299–313.

DINTENFASS, L. (1964b) Rheologic approach to thrombosis and atherosclerosis, *Angiology* **15**, 333–43.

DINTENFASS, L. (1965a) Viscosity of the packed red and white blood cells, *Exp. Molec. Path.* **4**, 597–605.

DINTENFASS, L. (1965b) A study in rheology of blood clotting in human subjects, *Proc. Fourth Int. Congr. on Rheol. 4, Symp. on Biorheol.*, ed. Copley, A. L., Interscience, New York, pp. 593–600.

DINTENFASS, L. (1967a) Rheology of blood in cardiovascular diseases. *Bibl. anat.* **9**, 525–31.

DINTENFASS, L. (1967b) Viscosity of blood at high hematocrits measured in microcapillary (parallel-plate) viscometers of $r = 3$–30 microns. (Abstract), *Biorheol.* **4**, 81–2.

DIX, F. S. and SCOTT BLAIR, G. W. (1940) On the flow of suspensions through narrow tubes, *J. appl. Phys.* **11**, 574–81.

DOLLERY, C. T., HENKIND, P., PATERSON, J. W. and RAMALHO, P. S. (1967) Circulatory changes following retinal embolism by glass microspheres. *Bibl. anat.* **9**, 112–5.

DOW, P., HAHN, P. F. and HAMILTON, W. F. (1946) The simultaneous transport of T-1824 and radio-active red cells through the heart and lungs, *Am. J. Physiol.* **147**, 493–9.

DUNAWAY, P. B. and LEWIS, L. L. (1965) Taxonomic relation of erythrocyte count, mean corpuscular volume and body weight in mammals, *Nature (London)*, **205**, 481–4.

ECKSTEIN, R. W., BOOK, D. and GREGG, D. E. (1941) Blood viscosity under different experimental conditions and its effect on blood flow, *Am. J. Physiol.* **135**, 772–5.

EHRLY, A. M. (1966) Wirkung von niedermolekülarem Dextran auf Erythrozyten-aggregate beim Sludgephänomen, *Med. Klin.* **61**, 989–92.

EINSTEIN, A. (1906) Eine neue Bestimmung der Moleküldimensionen, *Ann. Physik.* **19**, 289–306.

EIRICH, F. R. (1956) *Rheology*, vol. 1, Academic Press, New York.

ELIASSON, R. and SAMELIUS-BROBERG, U. (1965) The effect of dextran and some other colloids on the suspension stability of blood from different species, *Acta physiol. scand.* **64**, 245–50.

ENGESET, J., STALKER, A. L. and MATHESON, N. A. (1966) Effects of dextran 40 on erythrocyte aggregation, *Lancet* **1**, 1124–7.

ERICHSON, R. B. and CINTRON, J. R. (1966) Ultrastructural observations of platelet–fibrin interaction, *Proc. Fourth Europ. Conf. on Microcirc.*, Cambridge, Abstract 17.

ERSLEV, A. J. and ATWATER, J. (1963) The effect of mean corpuscular haemoglobin concentration on viscosity, *J. Lab. clin. Med.* **62**, 401–6.

EVANS, R. L. (1962) Pulsatile flow in vessels whose distensibility and size vary with site, *Physics Med. Biol.* **7**, 105–16.

EVANS, R. L., BERNSTEIN, E. F., JOHNSON, E. and RELLER, C. (1962) Mechanical properties of the living dog aorta, *Am. J. Physiol.* **202**, 619–21.

FAHRAEUS, R. (1929) The suspension stability of blood, *Physiol. Rev.* **9**, 241–74.

FAHRAEUS, R. (1958) The influence of the rouleau formation of the erythrocytes on the rheology of blood, *Acta med. scand.* **161**, 151–65.

FAHRAEUS, R. and LINDQVIST, T. (1931) The viscosity of the blood in narrow capillary tubes, *Am. J. Physiol.* **96**, 562–8.

FAWCETT, D. W. (1959) The fine structure of capillaries, arterioles and small arteries, *The Microcirculation*, ed. Reynolds, S. R. M. and Zweifach, B. W., University Press, Illinois, Urbana, pp. 1–27.

FOSTER, J. F. (1960) Plasma albumin. *The Plasma Proteins*, vol. 1, ed. Putman, F. W., Academic Press, New York, pp. 179–239.

FOURMAN, J. and MOFFAT, D. B. (1961) The effect of intra-arterial cushions on plasma skimming in small arteries, *J. Physiol.* **158**, 374–80.

FREDRICKSON, A. G. (1964) *Principles and Applications of Rheology*, Prentice-Hall, New Jersey.

FREIS, E. D., STANTON, J. R. and EMERSON, C. P. (1949) Estimation of relative velocities of plasma and red cells in the circulation of man. *Am. J. Physiol.* **157**, 153–7.

FREIS, E. D. and HEATH, W. C. (1964) Hydrodynamics of aortic blood flow, *Circulation Res.* **14**, 105–16.

FULTON, G. P., BERMAN, H. J., SLECHTA, R. F. and BROOKS, A. M. (1967) Rheological patterns in the microcirculation. (Abstract), *Biorheol.* **4**, 97–8.

FULTON, W. F. M. (1965) *The Coronary Arteries*, Thomas, Springfield.

FUNG, Y. C., ZWEIFACH, B. W. and INTAGLIETTA, M. (1966). Elastic environment of the capillary bed, *Circulation Res*. **19**, 441–61.

GELIN, L. E. (1961) Disturbance of the flow properties of blood and its counteraction in surgery, *Acta chir. scand*. **122**, 287–92.

GELIN, L. E. (1965) Rheological disturbances following tissue injury, *Proc. Fourth Int. Congr. on Rheol*. **4**, *Symp. on Biorheol*., ed. Copley, A. L., Interscience, New York, 299–315.

GELIN, L. E., RUDENSTAM, C. M. and ZEDERFELDT, B. (1965) The rheology of red cell suspensions, *Bibl. anat*. **7**, 368–75.

GELIN, L. E., BRUNIUS, U., FRITJOFSSON, A. and LEWIS, D. H. (1967) Hemodilution and kidney function during shock. *Bibl. anat*. **9.**, 311–20.

GIBSON, J. G., SELIGMAN, A. M., PEACOCK, W. C., AUB, J. C., FINE, J. and EVANS, R. D. (1946) The distribution of red cells and plasma in large and minute vessels of the normal dog determined by radio-active isotopes of iron and iodine, *J. clin. Invest*. **25**, 848–57.

GOLDSMITH, H. L. and MASON, S. G. (1961) Axial migration of particles in Poiseuille flow, *Nature* (*London*) **190**, 1095–6.

GOLDSMITH, H. L. and MASON, S. G. (1963) The flow of suspensions in tubes, *J. Colloid Sci*. **18**, 237–61.

GOLDSMITH, H. L. and MASON, S. G. (1965) Further comments on the radial migration of spheres in Poiseuille flow, *Biorheol*. **3**, 33–40.

GOLDSMITH, H. L. and MASON, S. G. (1967) The microrheology of dispersions. *Rheology*, vol. 4, ed. Eirich, F. R., Academic Press, New York.

GOLDSTEIN, S. (1938) *Modern Developments in Fluid Dynamics*, Vol. 1, Clarendon Press, Oxford.

GOODEVE, C. (1939) A general theory of thixotropy and viscosity, *Trans. Faraday Soc*. **35**, 342–58.

GORESKY, C. A. (1963) A linear method for determining liver sinusoidal and extravascular volumes, *Am. J. Physiol*. **204**, 626–40.

GREEN, H. D. (1944) Circulation: physical principles, *Medical Physics*, ed. Glasser, O., Year Book Med., Chicago, pp. 208–32.

GREENFIELD, A. D. M. (1962) Physiology of the venous system, *Blood Vessels and Lymphatics*, ed. Abramson, D. I., Academic Press, New York, pp. 197–207.

GREGERSON, M. I. (1966) Private communication.

GREGERSON, M. I. and ROOT, W. S. (1961) Hemorrhage and shock, *Medical Physiology*, 11th edn., ed. Bard, P., Mosby, St. Louis, pp. 283–97.

GREGERSON, M. I., PERIC, B., CHIEN, S., SINCLAIR, D., CHANG, C. and TAYLOR, H. (1965) Viscosity of blood at low shear rates, *Proc. Fourth Int. Congr. on Rheol*. **4**, *Symp. on Biorheol*., ed. Copley, A. L., Interscience, New York, pp. 613–28.

GREGERSON, M. I. and BRYANT, C. A. (1967) Studies on deformation of normal and abnormal red cells by microfiltration. (Abstract), *Biorheol*. **4**, 94.

GROOM, A. C. (1967) Transit times of cells and albumin through the vascular bed of skeletal muscle. (Abstract), *Biorheol*. **4**, 98.

GROTH, C. G. (1966) The effect of infused albumin and Rheomacrodex on factors governing the flow properties of human blood, *Acta chir. scand*. **131**, 290–7.

GROTH, C. G., LÖFSTRÖM, B., RYBECK, B. and THORSEN, G. (1964a) Effect of high and low molecular weight dextran on tissue oxygen tension, *Bibl. anat*. **4**, 174–8.

GROTH, C. G. and LÖFSTRÖM, B. (1964b) Conjunctival microscopy and erythrocyte sedimentation rate as methods for examining erythrocyte aggregation, *Bibl. anat*. **4**, 179–83.

GROTH, C. G. and MURUK, O. (1964c) Changes in blood plasma viscosity in experimentally induced erythrocyte aggregation, *Bibl. anat.* **7**, 385–9.

GROTH, C. G. and THORSEN, G. (1965) The effect of Rheomacrodex and Macrodex on factors governing the flow properties of blood, *Acta chir. scand.* **130**, 507–20.

GROTH, C. G., LÖFSTRÖM, B. and MURUK, O. (1966) The effect of infused thrombin on the tissue oxygen tension, *Acta chir. scand.* **132**, 1–14.

GUEST, M. M., BOND, T. P., COOPER, R. G. and DERRICK, J. R. (1963) Red blood cells: change in shape in capillaries, *Science* **142**, 1319–21.

GUYTON, A. C. (1961) *Textbook of Medical Physiology*, Saunders, Philadelphia.

GUYTON, A. C. (1963) *Circulatory Physiology; Cardiac Output and its Regulation*, Saunders, Philadelphia.

HADDY, F. J. (1962) Arterial and arteriolar systems II, *Blood Vessels and Lymphatics*, ed. Abramson, D. I., Academic Press, New York, pp. 61–6.

HALL, C. E. and SLAYTER, H. S. (1959) The fibrinogen molecule: its size, shape and mode of polymerization, *J. Biophys. Biochem. Cytology* **5**, 11–16.

HALL, W. M. (1932) Comments on the theory of horns, *J. acoust. Soc. Am.* **3**, 552–61.

HARDAWAY, R. M. (1967) Capillary blood flow and coagulation in shock. (Abstract), *Biorheol.* **4**, 101–2.

HARDUNG, V. (1962) Propagation of pulse waves in visco-elastic tubings, *Handbook on Physiology*. Sect. 2. Circulation, ed. Hamilton, W. F. and Dow, P., Am. Physiol. Soc., Washington, pp. 107–35.

HARKNESS, J. (1965) Measurement and clinical value of plasma viscosity, Rptd. by Whitmore, R. L. in Biorheological aspects of living microscopy, *Biorheol.* **3**, 41–2.

HARRIS, P. D. (1967) Quantification of capillary RBC flow. *Bibl. anat.* **9**, 155–9.

HARTERT, H. (1960) Thrombelastography, *Flow Properties of Blood*, ed. Copley, A. L. and Stainsby, G., Pergamon, London, pp. 186–96.

HARTERT, H. (1965) Clot retraction. Kinetics and correlation with the clotting process, *Proc. Fourth Int. Congr. on Rheol.* **4**, *Symp. on Biorheol.*, ed. Copley, A. L., Interscience, New York, pp. 571–80.

HARTERT, H. (1967) Behaviour of platelets in clot retraction. (Abstract), *Biorheol.* **4**, 86.

HAUROWITZ, F. (1961) The role of the blood plasma in bodily maintenance and repair, *Functions of the Blood*, ed. Macfarlane, R. G. and Robb-Smith, A. H. T., Academic Press, New York, pp. 527–602.

HAYNES, R. H. (1960) Physical basis of the dependence of blood viscosity on tube radius, *Am. J. Physiol.* **198**, 1193–1200.

HAYNES, R. H. and BURTON, A. C. (1959) Role of the non-Newtonian behaviour of blood in hemodynamics. *Am. J. Physiol.* **197**, 943–50.

HELPS, E. P. W. and MCDONALD, D. A. (1954) Observations on laminar flow in veins, *J. Physiol.* **124**, 631–9.

HERSHEY, D. and CHO, S. J. (1966) Blood flow in rigid tubes: thickness and slip velocity of plasma film at the wall, *J. appl. Physiol.* **21**, 27–32.

HIGGINBOTHAM, G. H., OLIVER, D. R. and WARD, S. G. (1958) Studies of the viscosity and sedimentation of suspensions. Part 4—capillary tube viscometry applied to stable suspensions of spherical particles, *Br. J. appl. Phys.* **9**, 372–7.

HIGHGATE, D. (1966) Particle migration in cone-plate viscometry of suspensions, *Nature (London)* **211**, 1390.

HILL, W. S. and POLLERI, J. O. (1964) Elementary hydrodynamic basis of an analog of the global blood circulation: congestive pulmonary failure, *Pulsatile Blood Flow*, ed. Attinger, E. O., McGraw-Hill, New York, pp. 407–21.

HINKE, J. A. M. and WILSON, M. L. (1962) A study of the elastic properties of a 550 μ artery *in vitro*, *Am. J. Physiol.* **203**, 1153–60.

HISSEN, W., SWANK, R. L., LINO, L. and SEAMAN, G. V. F. (1966) Physico-chemical changes in circulating blood on exsanguination or administration of histamine, *Surgery Gynec. Obstet.* **122**, 1003–14.

HOPPMANN, W. H. and BARONET, C. N. (1964) Flow generated by cone rotating in a liquid, *Nature (London)* **201**, 1205.

HORLOCK, J. A. (1962) Some experiments on the secondary flow in pipe bends, *Proc. Roy. Soc.* A, **234**, 335–46.

HOWE, J. T. and SHEAFFER, Y. S. (1966) *On the Dynamics of Capillaries and the Existence of Plasma Flow in the Pericapillary Lymph Space*, N.A.S.A. Tech. Note, NASA TN D-3497, 1966, 28 pp.

INTAGLIETTA, M. (1967) Evidence for a gradient of permeability in frog mesenteric capillaries. *Bibl. anat.* **2**, 465–8.

JACOBS, H. R. (1966) Meniscal resistance in tube viscometry, *Biorheol.* **3**, 117–40.

JAGER, G. N., WESTERHOF, N. and NOORDERGRAAF, A. (1965) Oscillatory flow impedance in electrical analogue of arterial system, *Circulation Res.* **16**, 121–33.

JEFFERY, G. B. (1922) The motion of ellipsoidal particles immersed in a viscous fluid, *Proc. Roy. Soc.* A, **102**, 161–79.

JEFFORDS, J. V. and KNISELY, M. H. (1956) Concerning the geometric shapes of arteries and arterioles; a contribution to the biophysics of health, disease and death, *Angiology* **7**, 105–36.

JEFFREY, R. C. and PEARSON, J. R. A. (1965) Particle motion in laminar vertical tube flow, *J. Fluid Mech.* **22**, 721–35.

JOLY, M. (1965) Contribution de la viscosimétrie à l'étude de la denaturation des proteines, *Biorheol.* **2**, 207–19.

JONES, A. L. (1966) On the flow of blood in a tube, *Biorheol.* **3**, 183–8.

KARNIS, A., GOLDSMITH, H. L. and MASON, S. G. (1965) *The Flow of Suspensions through Tubes. V. Concentrated Suspensions of Rigid Particles*, Tech. Rept. 432, Pulp and Paper Res. Inst., Canada.

KARNIS, A., GOLDSMITH, H. L. and MASON, S. G. (1966a) The flow of suspensions through tubes. V(b). Inertial effects, *Can. J. chem. Engng.* **44**, 181–93.

KARNIS, A. and MASON, S. G. (1966b) *The Flow of Suspensions through Tubes. VI. Meniscus Effects*, Tech. Rept. 450, Pulp and Paper Res. Inst., Canada.

KATCHALSKY, A., KEDEM, O., KLIBANSKY, C. and DE VRIES, A. (1960) Rheological considerations of the haemolysing red blood cell, *Flow Properties of Blood*, ed. Copley, A. L. and Stainsby, G., Pergamon, London, 155–69.

KAYE, G. W. C. and LABY, T. H. (1959) *Tables of Physical and Chemical Constants*, 12th edn., Longmans, London.

KIRK, J. E. (1962) Venous system, *Blood Vessels and Lymphatics*, ed. Abramson, D. I., Academic Press, New York, pp. 211–2.

KNISELY, M. H. (1951) An annotated bibliography on sludged blood, *Postgraduate Medicine* **10**, 15–93.

KNISELY, M. H. (1963) Experimental separation of quite different types of shock, *Israel J. exp. Med.* **11**, 147.

KNISELY, M. H. (1965) Intravascular erythrocyte aggregation (blood sludge), *Handbook of Physiology*, Sect. 2, Circulation, ed. Hamilton, W. F. and Dow, P., Am. Physiol. Soc., Washington, pp. 2249–92.

KNISELY, M. H., BLOCH, E. H., ELIOT, T. S. and WARNER, L. (1950) Sludged blood, *Trans. Am. ther. Soc.* **48**, 95–112.

KNISELY, W. H., MAHALEY, M. S. and JETT, H. H. (1958) Approximation of "total vascular space" and its distribution in three sizes of blood vessels in rats by plaster casts, *Circulation Res.* **6**, 20–5.

KNOX, C. K. (1962) An Experimental Investigation of the Steady Flow of a Viscous Fluid in Circular Branched Tubes, MS. thesis, Univ. of Minnesota.

KOCHEN, J. A. (1965) Flow properties of hemoglobin in the hemolysing red cell, *Proc. Fourth Int. Congr. on Rheol. 4, Symp. on Biorheol.*, ed. Copley, A. L., Interscience, New York, pp. 193–9.

KOCHEN, J. A. (1967) Visco-elastic properties of the red cell membrane. (Abstract), *Biorheol.* **4,** 90–1.

KOK, D'A. (1966) Studies of the viscosity of serum in disease states, using a capillary viscometer, *Biorheol.* **3,** 216–7.

KREUZER, F. (1950) Investigations concerning the viscosity of blood serum, *Helv. physiol. pharmac. Acta* **8,** 486–504.

KROGH, A. (1922) *The Anatomy and Physiology of Capillaries,* University Press, Yale, New Haven.

KROGH, A. (1959) *The Anatomy and Physiology of Capillaries,* Hafner, New York.

KÜMIN, K. (1949) Inaugural dissertation, Univ. of Bern.

KURLAND, G. S., BROWN, S., TOUSIGNANT, P. and CHARM, S. (1967) Studies of blood flow in a living vessel. (Abstract), *Biorheol.* **4,** 97.

KURODA, K., MISHIRO, Y. and WADA, I. (1958) Relation between the viscosity of erythrocyte suspension and the shape of erythrocyte, *Tokushima J. exp. Med.* **4,** 73–82.

KURODA, K. and FUJINO, M. (1963) On the cause of increase in light transparency of erythrocyte suspensions in flow, *Biorheol.* **1,** 167–82.

KURODA, K. and FUJINO, M. (1964) Fundamental conditions for measuring the "streaming transparency" of erythrocyte suspension, *Biorheol.* **2,** 97–101.

LAMB, H. (1932) *Hydrodynamics,* 6th edn., University Press, Cambridge.

LAMBERT, J. W. (1958) On the nonlinearities of flow in nonrigid tubes, *J. Franklin Inst.* **266,** 83–102.

LANDIS, E. M. and PAPPENHEIMER, J. R. (1963) Exchanges of substances through the capillary walls, *Handbook of Physiology,* Sect. 2, Circulation, ed. Hamilton, W. F. and Dow, P., Am. Physiol. Soc., Washington, pp. 961–1034.

LAWTON, R. W. (1955) Measurement of the elasticity and damping of isolated aortic strips of the dog, *Circulation Res.* **3,** 403–8.

LEAROYD, B. M. and TAYLOR, M. G. (1966) Alterations with age in the visco-elastic properties of human arterial walls, *Circulation Res.* **18,** 278–92.

LEE, W. H. (1966) The significance of apparent blood viscosity in circulating hemodynamic behaviour, *Proc. Fourth Europ. Conf. on Microcirc., Cambridge,* Abstract 36.

LEHMANN, H. and HUNTSMAN, R. G. (1961) The evolution of the human red cell, *Functions of the Blood,* ed. Macfarlane, R. G. and Robb-Smith, A. H. T., Academic Press, London, pp. 73–148.

LEITH, W. C. (1966) Cavitation effects in the blood circulatory system, *Biomedical Fluid Mech. Symp., Colorado,* Am. Soc. Mech. Engrs., pp. 110–21.

LEROUX, M. E. (1965) La propriété thrombodynamique du caillot, *Proc. Fourth Int. Congr. on Rheol. 4, Symp. on Biorheol.*, ed. Copley, A. L., Interscience, New York, pp. 549–69.

LEVICH, V. G. (1962) *Physicochemical Hydrodynamics,* Prentice-Hall, New Jersey.

LIGHTHILL, M. J. (1966) Initial development of diffusion in Poiseuille flow, *J. Inst. Math. Applic. (G.B.)* **2,** 97–108.

LOVE, A. E. H. (1927) *A Treatise on Mathematical Elasticity,* 3rd edn. University Press, Cambridge.

LUFT, J. H. (1964) Fine structure of the vascular wall, *Evolution of the Athero-sclerotic Plaque*, ed. Jones, R. J., University Press, Chicago, pp. 3–14.

MACFARLANE, R. G. (1960) The blood coagulation system, *The Plasma Proteins*, vol. 2, ed. Putnam, F. W., Academic Press, London, pp. 137–81.

MACFARLANE, R. G. (1961) The reaction of the blood to injury, *Functions of the Blood*, ed. Macfarlane, R. G. and Robb-Smith, A. H. T., Academic Press, London, pp. 303–47.

MADOW, B. and BLOCH, E. H. (1956) The effect of erythrocyte aggregation on the rheology of blood, *Angiology* 7, 1–15.

MAGGIO, E. (1965) *Microhemocirculation*, Thomas, Springfield.

MAUDE, A. D. (1960) The viscosity of a suspension of spheres, *J. Fluid Mech.* 7, 230–6.

MAUDE, A. D. and WHITMORE, R. L. (1956) The wall effect and the viscometry of suspensions, *Br. J. appl. Phys.* 7, 98–102.

MAUDE, A. D. and WHITMORE, R. L. (1958) Theory of the flow of blood in narrow tubes, *J. appl. Physiol.* 12, 105–13.

MAUDE, A. D. and WALTERS, K. (1964) Approximate theory for oscillating experiments with a cone and plate viscometer, *Nature (London)* 201, 913–4.

MAYER, G. A. and KISS, O. (1965) Blood viscosity and *in vitro* anticoagulants, *Am. J. Physiol.* 208, 795–7.

MAYER, G. A., FRIDRICH, J., NEWELL, J. and SZIVEK, J. (1966) Plasma components and blood viscosity, *Biorheol.* 3, 177–82.

MAYERSON, H. S. (1962) Microcirculation, *Blood Vessels and Lymphatics*, ed. Abramson, D. I., Academic Press, New York, pp. 157–91.

McDONALD, D. A. (1960a) The velocity profiles of pulsatile blood flow, *Flow Properties of Blood*, ed. Copley, A. L. and Stainsby, G., Pergamon, London, pp. 84–95.

McDONALD, D. A. (1960b) *Blood Flow in Arteries*, Arnold, London.

McDONALD, D. A. and GESSNER, U. (1967) Wave propagation in visco-elastic arteries. (Abstract), *Biorheol.* 4, 73.

McMILLAN, G. C. (1962) Abnormalities of the venous system, *Blood Vessels and Lymphatics*, ed. Abramson, D. I., Academic Press, New York, pp. 680–8.

MEISELMAN, H. J. and MERRILL, E. W. (1967) The effect of the addition of dextran on the rheological properties of blood. (Abstract), *Biorheol.* 4, 896.

MEISNER, J. E. and RUSHMER, R. F. (1963) Eddy formation and turbulence in flowing liquids, *Circulation Res.* 12, 455–63.

MERRILL, E. W. and WELLS, R. E. (1961) Flow properties of biological fluids, *Appl. Mech. Rev.* 14, 663–73.

MERRILL, E. W., COKELET, G. C., BRITTEN, A. and WELLS, R. E. (1963a) Non-Newtonian rheology of human blood—effect of fibrinogen deduced by "subtraction", *Circulation Res.* 13, 48–55.

MERRILL, E. W., GILLILAND, E. R., COKELET, G., SHIN, H., BRITTEN, A. and WELLS, R. E. (1963b) Rheology of human blood—effects of temperature and hematocrit level, *Biophys. J.* 3, 199–213.

MERRILL, E. W., GILLILAND, E. R., MARGETTS, W. G. and HATCH, F. T. (1964) Rheology of human blood and hyperlipemia, *J. appl. Physiol.* 19, 493–6.

MERRILL, E. W., BENIS, A. M., GILLILAND, E. R., SHERWOOD, T. K. and SALZMAN, E. W. (1965a) Pressure-flow relations of human blood in hollow fibres at low flow rates, *J. appl. Physiol.* 20, 954–67.

MERRILL, E. W., MARGETTS, W. G., COKELET, G. R., BRITTEN, A., SALZMAN, E. W., PENNELL, R. B. and MELIN, M. (1965b) Influence of plasma proteins on the rheology of human blood, *Proc. Fourth Int. Congr. on Rheol. 4, Symp. on Biorheol.*, ed. Copley, A. L., Interscience, New York, pp. 601–11.

182 REFERENCES

MERRILL, E. W., GILLILAND, E. R., LEE, T. S. and SALZMAN, E. W. (1966) Blood rheology: effect of fibrinogen deduced by addition, *Circulation Res.* **18**, 437–46.

MERRINGTON, A. C. (1949) *Viscometry*, Arnold, London.

MICHAELS, A. S. and BOLGER, J. C. (1962) The plastic flow behaviour of flocculated kaolin suspensions, *Ind. Engng. Chem.-Fundls.* **1**, 153–62.

MITCHELL, J. R. A. and SCHWARTZ, C. J. (1965) *Arterial Disease*, Blackwell, London.

MOFFAT, D. B. (1965) The distribution of red blood cells in the renal cortex, *Clin. Sci.* **28**, 125–30.

MOON, V. H. (1944) Shock and haemorrhage, *Medical Physics*, ed. Glasser, O., Year Book Med., Chicago, 1415–20.

MONRO, P. A. G. (1963) The appearance of cell-free plasma and grouping of red blood cells in normal circulation, *Biorheol.* **1**, 239–46.

MONRO, P. A. G. (1964) The deformation of red cells and groups of cells in blood flowing in small blood vessels, *Bibl. anat.* **7**, 376–82.

MORECI, A. P. and FARBER, E. M. (1962) Cutaneous circulation, *Blood Vessels and Lymphatics*, ed. Abramson, D. I., Academic Press, New York, pp. 489–94.

MORELAND, C. (1963) Viscosity of suspensions of coal in mineral oil. *Can. J. chem. Engng.* **41**, 24–8.

MORGAN, B. C., ABEL, F. L., MULLINS, G. L. and GUNTHEROTH, W. G. (1966a) Flow patterns in cavae, pulmonary artery, pulmonary vein and aorta of intact dogs, *Am. J. Physiol.* **210**, 903–9.

MORGAN, B. C., DILLARD, D. H. and GUNTHEROTH, W. G. (1966b) Effect of cardiac and respiratory cycle on pulmonary vein flow, pressure and diameter, *J. appl. Physiol.* **21**, 1276–80.

MORKIN, E., LEVINE, R. and FISHMAN, A. P. (1964) Pulmonary capillary flow pulse and the site of pulmonary vasoconstriction in the dog, *Circulation Res.* **15**, 146–60.

MORKIN, E., COLLINS, J. A., GOLDMAN, H. S. and FISHMAN, A. P. (1965) Patterns of blood flow in the pulmonary veins of the dog, *J. appl. Physiol.* **20**, 1118–28.

MÜLLER, A. (1936) *Abhandlungen zur Mechanik der Flüssigkeiten, I*, Univ. of Freibourg.

MÜLLER, A. (1948) On the pressure relationships in blood vessels especially in the capillaries, *Helv. physiol. pharmac. Acta* **6**, 181–95.

MURPHY, J. R. (1967) The effect of pH and temperature on rheological properties of the erythrocyte. (Abstract), *Biorheol.* **4**, 91–2.

MUSTARD, J. F., MURPHY, E. A., ROWSELL, H. C. and DOWNIE, H. G. (1962) Factors influencing thrombus formation *in vivo*, *Amer. J. Med.* **33**, 621–47.

NALLY, M. C. (1965) The oscillatory motion of an elastico-viscous liquid in a cone and plate viscometer, *Br. J. appl. Phys.* **16**, 1023–31.

NAWAB, M. A. and MASON, S. G. (1958) The viscosity of dilute suspensions of threadlike particles, *J. phys. Chem. Ithaca.* **62**, 1248–53.

NICHOL, J. T. (1955) The effect of cholesterol feeding on the distensibility of the isolated thoracic aorta of the rabbit, *Can. J. Biochem. Physiol.* **33**, 507–16.

NISHIMURA, J. and OKA, S. (1965) The steady flow of a viscous fluid through a tapered tube, *J. phys. Soc. Japan.* **20**, 449–53.

NOORDERGRAAF, A., VERDOUW, P. D., VAN BRUMMELEN, A. G. W. and WIEGEL, F. W. (1964) Analog of the arterial bed, *Pulsatile Blood Flow*, ed. Attinger, E. O., McGraw-Hill, New York, pp. 373–87.

NORRIS, R. (1869) On the laws and principles concerned in the aggregation of blood corpuscles both within and without the vessels, *Proc. Roy. Soc.* A **171**, 429–36.

OBIAKOR, E. K. and WHITMORE, R. L. (1964) The effect of stepwise flocculation on the rheology of a kaolin clay suspension, *J. Oil Colour Chem. Ass.* **47**, 334–45.

OKA, S. (1960) The principles of rheometry, *Rheology*, vol. 3, ed. Eirich, F. R., Academic Press, New York.

OKA, S. (1964) The steady slow motion of a viscous fluid through a tapered tube, *J. phys. Soc. Japan.* **19**, 1481–4.

OKA, S. (1965) Theoretical considerations of the flow of blood through a capillary, *Proc. Fourth Int. Congr. on Rheol. 4, Symp. on Biorheol.*, ed. Copley, A. L., Interscience, New York, pp. 89–102.

OKA, S. (1967) Theoretical approach to the effect of wall surface condition in hemorheology. (Abstract), *Biorheol.* **4**, 75–6.

OLDENDORF, W. H., KITANO, M., SHIMIZU, S. and OLDENDORF, S. Z. (1965) Hematocrit of the human cranial blood pool, *Circulation Res.* **17**, 532–9.

OLDROYD, J. G. (1949) The interpretation of observed pressure gradients in flow through tubes, *J. Colloid Sci.* **4**, 333–5.

OLIVER, D. R. and WARD, S. G. (1953) Relationship between relative viscosity and volume concentration of stable suspensions of spherical particles, *Nature (London)* **171**, 396–7.

OLSON, R. M. (1964) *In vivo* blood viscosity and hinderance, *Am. J. Physiol.* **206**, 955–61.

PAI, SH. I. (1956) *Viscous Flow Theory*, vol. 1, Laminar Flow, van Nostrand, Princeton.

PALMER, A. A. (1959) A study of blood flow in minute vessels of the pancreatic region of the rat with reference to intermittent corpuscular flow in individual arteries, *Q. Jl. exp. Physiol.* **44**, 149–59.

PALMER, A. A. (1965a) Plasma skimming in human blood flowing through branching glass capillary channels, *Proc. Fourth Int. Congr. on Rheol. 4, Symp. on Biorheol.*, ed. Copley, A. L., Interscience, New York, 245–53.

PALMER, A. A. (1965b) Axial drift of cells and partial plasma skimming in blood flowing through glass slits, *Am. J. Physiol.* **209**, 1115–22.

PALMER, A. A. (1967a) Platelet and leucocyte skimming. *Bibl. anat.* **9**, 300–3.

PALMER, A. A. (1967b) Some aspects of plasma skimming. (Abstract), *Biorheol.* **4**, 88.

PAPPENHEIMER, J. R. and KINTER, W. B. (1956) Hematocrit ratio of blood within mammalian kidney and its significance for renal hemodynamics, *Am. J. Physiol.* **185**, 377–90.

PASSOW, H. (1964) Iron and water permeability of the red blood cell, *The Red Blood Cell*, ed. Bishop, C. and Surgenor, D. M., Academic Press, New York, pp. 71–145.

PATEL, D. J., GREENFIELD, J. C. and FRY, D. L. (1964) *In vivo* pressure–length–radius relationship of certain blood vessels in man and dog, *Pulsatile Blood Flow*, ed. Attinger, E. O., McGraw-Hill, New York, pp. 293–302.

PATEL, D. J., GREENFIELD, J. C., AUSTEN, W. G., MORROW, A. G. and FRY, D. L. (1965) Pressure-flow relationships in the ascending aorta and femoral artery of man, *J. appl. Physiol.* **20**, 459–63.

PATERSON, J. C. (1962) Deep venous thrombosis, *Blood Vessels and Lymphatics*, ed. Abramson, D. I., Academic Press, New York, pp. 688–98.

PATERSON, J. W., DOLLERY, C. T., RAMALHO, P. S. and KOHNER, E. M. (1967) The effects of platelet aggregates on the retinal microcirculation. *Bibl. anat.* **9**, 85–91.

Pease, D. C. (1962) Fine structure of elastic arteries, *Blood Vessels and Lymphatics*, ed. Abramson, D. I., Academic Press, New York, pp. 12–8.

Pennell, R. B. (1964) Composition of normal human red cells, *The Red Blood Cell*, ed. Bishop, C. and Surgenor, D. M., Academic Press, New York, pp. 29–69.

Perel'man, I. M. (1965) Near-wall slipping of blood in capillaries, *Kolloidnyi Zhurnal*. 27, 422. (*Rheology Abstracts* 652/65).

Peric, B. (1963) Viscosity of the blood at low shear rates, *Israel J. exp. Med.* 11, 139.

Petermann, M. L. (1960) Alterations in plasma protein patterns in disease, *The Plasma Proteins*, vol. 2, ed. Putnam, F. W., Academic Press, New York, pp. 309–43.

Peterson, L. H. (1962) Properties and behaviour of living vascular wall, *Physiol. Rev.* 42, 309–24.

Peterson, L. H. (1964) Vessel wall stress–strain relationship, *Pulsatile Blood Flow*, ed. Attinger, E. O., McGraw-Hill, New York, pp. 263–71.

Peterson, L. H. (1966) Physical factors which influence vascular caliber and blood flow, *Circulation Res.*, Suppt. 1, 18, I3–I13.

Peterson, L. H., Jensen, R. E. and Parnell, J. (1960) Mechanical properties of arteries *in vivo*, *Circulation Res.* 8, 622–39.

Phelps, R. A. and Putnam, F. W. (1960) Chemical composition and molecular parameters of purified plasma proteins, *The Plasma Proteins*, ed. Putnam, F. W., Academic Press, New York, pp. 143–78.

Phibbs, R. H. (1966) Distribution of leukocytes in blood flowing through arteries, *Am. J. Physiol.* 210, 919–25.

Phibbs, R. H. (1967) Orientation and distribution of erythrocytes in blood flowing through medium-sized arteries. (Abstract), *Biorheol.* 4, 97.

Philip, J. R. (1963) A theory of dispersal during laminar flow in tubes, *Austr. J. Phys.* 16, 287–310.

Ponder, E. (1948) *Hemolysis and Related Phenomena*, Churchill, London.

Ponder, E. (1966) Compression of human red cells during centrifuging, *Nature (London)* 210, 527.

Prandtl, L. (1952) *Essentials of Fluid Dynamics*, Blackie, London.

Prandtl, L. and Tietjens, O. G. (1934) *Applied Hydro and Aeromechanics*, McGraw-Hill, New York.

Pringle, R., Walder, D. N. and Weaver, J. P. (1965) Blood viscosity and Reynaud's disease, *Lancet* 1, 1086–9.

Prothero, J. and Burton, A. C. (1962a) The physics of blood flow in capillaries: II. The capillary resistance to flow, *Biophys. J.* 2, 199–212.

Prothero, J. and Burton, A. C. (1962b) The physics of blood flow in capillaries: III. The pressure required to deform erythrocytes, *Biophys. J.* 2, 213–22.

Putnam, F. W. (1960) Abnormal serum globulins, *The Plasma Proteins*, vol. 2, ed. Putnam, F. W., Academic Press, New York, pp. 345–406.

Rand, P. W., Lacombe, E., Hunt, H. E. and Austin, W. H. (1964a) Viscosity of normal human blood under normothermic and hypothermic conditions, *J. appl. Physiol.* 19, 117–22.

Rand, R. P. and Burton, A. C. (1963) Area and volume changes in hemolysis of single erythrocytes, *J. cell. comp. Physiol.* 61, 245–53.

Rand, R. P. and Burton, A. C. (1964b) Mechanical properties of the red cell membrane, *Biophys. J.* 4, 115–35.

Ranke, O. F. (1934) Die Dämpfung der Pulswelle und die innere Reibung der Arterienwand, *Z. Biol.* 95, 179–204.

RASHEVSKY, N. (1960) *Mathematical Biophysics*, vol. 2, 3rd edn., Dover, New York, p. 295.

REES, S. B., SIMON, L., PELTIER, G. A., BALODIMOS, M., GLEASON, R., MARBLE, A. and MERRILL, E. W. (1967) Hemorheologic studies during the progression and remission of diabetic retinopathy. (Abstract), *Biorheol.* 4, 102.

REEVE, E. B., GREGERSON, M. I., ALLEN, T. H., SEAR, H. and WALCOTT, W. W. (1953) Effects of alteration in blood volume and venous hematocrit in splenectomized dogs on estimates of total blood volume with P^{32} and T-1824, *Am. J. Physiol.* 175, 204–10.

REINER, M. (1960) *Deformation, Strain and Flow*, Lewis, London.

REINER, M. and SCOTT BLAIR, G. W. (1959) The flow of the blood through narrow tubes, *Nature (London)* 184, 354.

RHODIN, J. A. G. (1962) Fine structure of vascular walls in mammals, *Physiol. Rev.* 42, Suppt. 5 48–81.

RHODIN, J. A. G. (1967a) The ultrastructure of mammalian arterioles and precapillary sphincters. *J. Ultrastructure Res.* 18, 181–223.

RHODIN, J. A. G. (1967b) Ultrastructure of precapillary and postcapillary vessels. *Bibl. anat.* 9, 154.

RICHARDSON, E. G. (1950) *Dynamics of Real Fluids*, Arnold, London, p.119.

ROACH, M. and BURTON, A. C. (1957) The reason for the shape of the distensibility curves of arteries, *Can. J. Biochem. Physiol.* 35, 681–90.

ROACH, M. R. and BURTON, A. C. (1959) The effect of age on the elasticity of human arteries, *Can. J. Biochem. Physiol.* 37, 557–69.

RODBARD, S. (1962) Arterial and arteriolar systems, I. *Blood Vessels and Lymphatics*, ed. Abramson, D. I., Academic Press, New York, pp. 31–61.

ROSCOE, R. (1953) Suspensions, *Flow Properties of Disperse Systems*, ed. Hermans, J. J., North Holland, Amsterdam, pp. 1–38.

ROSENBLATT, G., STOKES, J. and BASSETT, D. R. (1965) Whole blood viscosity-hematocrit and serum lipid levels in normal subjects and patients with coronary heart disease, *J. Lab. clin. Med.* 65, 202–11.

ROSTON, S. (1964) The arterial circulation of the heart, *Bull. math. Biophys.* 26, 113–9.

ROUSE, H. (1946) *Elementary Mechanics of Fluids*, Wiley, New York.

ROWLANDS, S., GROOM, A. C. and THOMAS, H. W. (1965) The difference in circulation times between erythrocytes and plasma *in vivo, Proc. Fourth Int. Congr. on Rheol. 4, Symp. on Biorheol.*, ed. Copley, A. L., Interscience, New York, pp. 371–9.

ROZENBERG, M. C. and DINTENFASS, L. (1964) Thrombus formation *in vitro*, *Aust. J. exp. Biol. med. Sci.* 42, 109–15.

ROZENBERG, M. C. and DINTENFASS, L. (1966) Platelet aggregation in the variable-frequency thromboviscometer, *Nature (London)* 211, 525–6.

RUBINOW, S. I. and KELLER, J. B. (1967) A hydrodynamic theory of the circulatory system. (Abstract) *Biorheol.* 4, 79–80.

RUDINGER, G. (1966) Review of current mathematical methods for the analysis of blood flow, *Biomedical Fluid Mech. Symp., Colorado*, Am. Soc. Mech. Engrs., pp. 1–33.

RUTGERS, R. (1962) Relative viscosity of suspensions of rigid spheres in New tonian liquids, *Rheol. Acta* 2, 202–10.

RUTTY, D. A. (1965) A mechanism to limit platelet aggregation *in vivo*, *Nature (London)* 206, 1263.

SACKS, A. H. and TICKNER, E. G. (1967) Laminar flow regimes for rigid-sphere suspensions. (Abstract) *Biorheol.* 4, 84.

SADRON, CH. (1953) Dilute solutions of impenetrable rigid particles, *Flow Properties of Disperse Systems*, ed. Hermans, J. J., North Holland, Amsterdam, pp. 131–98.

SAFFMAN, P. G. (1965) The lift on a small sphere in a slow shear flow, *J. Fluid Mech.* **22**, 385–400.

SANDERS, A. G. and MACFARLANE, R. D. (1966) Reactions to injury of small blood vessels, *Proc. Fourth Europ. Conf. on Microcirc., Cambridge*, Abstract F.3.

SAUNDERS, E. A. and KNISELY, M. H. (1954) Living mesenteric terminal arterioles before and immediately after embolization and comparison of internal diameters, *A.M.A. Arch. Pathol.* **58**, 309–44.

SCHERAGA, H. A. (1955) Non-Newtonian behaviour of solutions of ellipsoidal particles, *J. Chem. Phys.* **23**, 1526–32.

SCHOFIELD, R. K. and SCOTT BLAIR, G. W. (1930) The influence of the proximity of a solid wall on the consistency of viscous and plastic materials, *J. phys. Chem. Ithaca* **34**, 248–62.

SCHUMANN, J. and FREITAG, V. (1964) Intravascular aggregation of erythrocytes in human skin capillaries, *Bibl. anat.* **7**, 194–9.

SCOTT BLAIR, G. W. (1958) The importance of the sigma phenomenon in the study of the flow of blood, *Rheol. Acta* **1**, 123–6.

SCOTT BLAIR, G. W. (1960) Rheology of blood coagulation, *Flow Properties of Blood*, ed. Copley, A. L. and Stainsby, G., Pergamon, London, pp. 172–83.

SCOTT BLAIR, G. W. and BURNETT, J. (1960) Preliminary experiments on the rheology of bovine blood-clot, *Kolloidzeitschrift* **168**, 98–101.

SEAMAN, G. V. F. (1967) The role of electrical charge in the suspension stability and flow properties of red cell suspensions. (Abstract), *Biorheol.* **4**, 95.

SEAMAN, G. V. F. and UHLENBRUCK, G. (1963) The surface structure of erythrocytes from some animal species, *Archs. Biochem. Biophys.* **100**, 493–502.

SEAMAN, G. V. F. and PETHICA, B. A. (1964) A comparison of the electrophoretic characteristics of the human normal and sickle erythrocyte, *Biochem. J.* **90**, 573–8.

SEAMAN, G. V. F. and COOK, G. M. W. (1965a) Modification of the electrophoretic behaviour of the erythrocyte by chemical and enzymatic methods, *Cell Electrophoresis*, ed. Ambrose, E. J., Churchill, London, pp. 48–65.

SEAMAN, G. V. F., HISSEN, W., LINO, L. and SWANK, R. L. (1965b) Physicochemical changes in blood arising from dextran infusions, *Clin. Sci.* **29**, 293–304.

SEAMAN, G. V. F. and SWANK, R. L. (1967) The influence of electrokinetic charge and deformability of the red blood cell on the flow properties of its suspensions, *Biorheol.* **4**, 47–9.

SEGRE, G. and SILBERBERG, A. (1962) Behaviour of macroscopic rigid spheres in Poiseuille flow, *J. Fluid Mech.* **14**, 115–35, 136–57.

SEYMOUR, B. (1967) Pulsatile flow in the larger arteries. (Abstract), *Biorheol.* **4**, 78–9.

SHORTHOUSE, B. O. and HUTCHINSON, M. T. (1967) Investigation into the viscoelasticity of cell free plasma using the biorheogoniometer. *Bibl. anat.* **9**, 232–9.

SILBERBERG, A. (1966) The tubular pinch effect in the circulation of blood, *Biorheol.* **4**, 29–30.

SILBERBERG, A. (1967) Flow and interaction of particles in tubes. (Abstract), *Biorheol* **4**, 82–3.

SIMHA, R. (1940) The influence of Brownian movement on the viscosity of solutions, *J. phys. Chem. Ithaca* **44**, 25–34.

SKOVBORG, F., NIELSEN, A. V., SCHLICHTKRULL, J. and DITZEL, J. (1966) Blood viscosity in diabetic patients, *Lancet* 1, 129–31.

SKOVBORG, F., NIELSEN, A. V., SCHLICHTKRULL, J. and DITZEL, J. (1967) Further studies of the blood viscosity in diabetic patients, *Bibl. anat.* 9, 508.

SLEZKIN, N. A. (1955) *Dynamics of Viscous Incompressible Fluid*, Gos. Izdat. Tekh.-Teor. Lit., Moscow.

SNELL, R. E., CLEMENTS, J. M., PATEL, D. J., FRY, D. L. and LUCHSINGER, P. C. (1965) Instantaneous blood flow in the human aorta, *J. appl. Physiol.* 20, 691–5.

SOBIN, S. S. (1966) The architecture and function of the microvasculature, *Biomechanics*, Am. Soc. Mech. Engrs., New York.

SONG, C., CHARM, S. and KURLAND, G. (1965) Energy losses for blood flowing through tapered tubes and curved tubes, (Abstract only), *Proc. Fourth Int. Congr. on Rheol. 4, Symp. on Biorheol.*, ed. Copley, A. L., Interscience, New York, p. 255.

SPENCER, M. P. and DENISON, A. B. (1963) Pulsatile blood flow in the vascular system, *Handbook of Physiology*, Sect. 2, Circulation, ed. Hamilton, W. F. and Dow, P., Am. Physiol. Soc., Washington, pp. 839–64.

STALKER, A. L., ENGESET, J. and MATHESON, N. A. (1966) Leucocyte impaction and erythrocyte flow in arterioles, *Proc. Fourth Europ. Conf. on Microcirc., Cambridge*, Abstract F.4.

STEHBENS, W. E. (1960) Turbulence of blood flow in the vascular system of man, *Flow Properties of Blood*, ed. Copley, A. L. and Stainsby, G., Pergamon, London, pp. 137–40.

STEHBENS, W. E. (1967a) Aspects of blood flow and platelet agglutination. (Abstract), *Biorheol.* 4, 85.

STEHBENS, W. E. (1967b) Early intravascular platelet agglutination. *Bibl. anat.* 9, 82–4.

STEWART, G. J. (1967) Drug-induced changes in platelet ultrastructure, *Bibl. anat.* 9, 76–9.

STONE, H. (1964) Private communication.

STREETER, V. L., KEITZER, W. F. and BOHR, D. F. (1963) Pulsatile pressure and flow through distensible vessels, *Circulation Res.* 13, 3–20.

STRUMIA, M. M. (1964) Historical introduction, *The Red Blood Cell*, ed. Bishop, C. and Surgenor, D. M., Academic Press, New York, pp. 1–28.

STRUMIA, M. M. and PHILLIPS, M. (1963) Effect of red cell factors on the relative viscosity of whole blood, *Am. J. clin. Path.* 39, 464–74.

SWANK, R. L. (1954) Effect of high fat feedings on viscosity of the blood, *Science* 120, 427–8.

SWANK, R. L. (1956) Effect of fat on blood viscosity in dogs, *Circulation Res.* 4, 579–85.

SWANK, R. (1958) Suspension stability of blood after injections of dextran, *J. appl. Physiol.* 12, 125–8.

SWANK, R. L. (1959) Changes in blood of dogs and rabbits by high fat intake, *Am. J. Physiol.* 196, 473–7.

SWANK, R. L. (1962) Adhesiveness of platelets and leukocytes during acute exsanguination, *Am. J. Physiol.* 202, 261–4.

SWANK, R. L., ROTH, J. G. and JANSEN, J. (1964) Screen filtration pressure method and adhesiveness and aggregation of blood cells, *J. appl. Physiol.* 19, 340–6.

SWANK, R. L. and DAVIS, E. (1966a) Blood cell aggregation and screen filtration pressure, *Circulation* 33, 617–24.

SWANK, R. L., SEAMAN, G. V. F., HISSEN, W. and LINO, L. (1966b) Physicochemical changes in blood induced by trauma, *Surgery Gynec. Obstet.* 123, 251–9.

TANFORD, C. (1965) *Physical Chemistry of Macromolecules*, Wiley, New York.

TARG, S. M. (1951) *Basic Problems of the Theory of Laminar Flow*, Gos. Izdat. Tekh-Teor. Lit., Moscow.

TAYLOR, C. B. (1962) Arteriosclerosis; gross changes, *Blood Vessels and Lymphatics*, ed. Abramson, D. I., Academic Press, New York, pp. 572–6.

TAYLOR, H. M., CHIEN, S., GREGERSON, M. I. and LUNDBERG, J. L. (1965) Comparison of viscosity of suspensions of plastic spheres and human blood cells, *Nature (London)* **207**, 77–8.

TAYLOR, M. G. (1955) The flow of blood in narrow tubes II. The axial stream and its formation, as determined by changes in optical density, *Aust. J. exp. Biol. med. Sci.* **33**, 1–16.

TAYLOR, M. G. (1964) Wave travel in arteries and the design of the cardio-vascular system, *Pulsatile Blood Flow*, ed. Attinger, E. O., McGraw-Hill, New York, pp. 343–67.

TAYLOR, M. G. (1966a) An introduction to some recent developments in arterial haemodynamics, *Aust. Ann. Med.* **15**, 71–96.

TAYLOR, M. G. (1966b) The input impedance of an assembly of randomly branching elastic tubes, *Biophys. J.* **6**, 29–51.

TAYLOR, M. G. (1967) The influence of the viscous properties of blood and the arterial wall upon the input impedance of the arterial system, (Abstract), *Biorheol.* **4**, 79.

TAYLOR, M. G. and ROBERTSON, J. S. (1954) The flow of blood in narrow tubes. I. A capillary microphotometer: an apparatus for measuring the optical density of flowing blood, *Aust. J. exp. Biol. med. Sci.* **32**, 721–32.

TEITEL, P. (1965) Disk-sphere transformation and plasticity alteration of red blood cells, *Nature (London)* **206**, 409–10.

TEXON, M. (1960) The hemodynamic concept of atherosclerosis, *Bull. N.Y. Acad. Med.* **36**, 263–71.

THOMAS, H. W. (1962) The wall effect in capillary instruments, *Biorheol.* **1**, 41–56.

THOMAS, H. W. (1965) On the difference between the clearance curves of labelled red cells and labelled plasma from the circulatory bed of the heart and lung, *Biorheol.* **3**, 36–40.

THOMAS, H. W., FRENCH, R. J., GROOM, A. C. and ROWLANDS, S. (1965) The flow of red cell suspensions through narrow tubes: the (extracorporeal) determination of the difference in mean velocities of red cells and their suspending phase, *Proc. Fourth Int. Congr. on Rheol.* **4**, *Symp. on Biorheol.*, ed. Copley, A. L., Interscience, New York, pp. 381–91.

THOMAS, R. H. and WALTERS, K. (1963) On the flow of an elasticoviscous liquid in a curved pipe under a pressure gradient, *J. Fluid Mech.* **16**, 228–42.

THOMPSON, H. K. (1964) Private communication.

THORSEN, G. and HINT, H. (1950) Aggregation, sedimentation and intravascular sludging of erythrocytes, *Acta. chir. scand. Suppt.* **154**, 1–50.

TIMM, C. (1942) Der Strömungsverlauf in einem Modell der menschlichen Aorta, *Z. Biol.* **101**, 79–99.

TULLIS, J. L. (1953) The platelets of human blood, *Blood Cells and Plasma Proteins*, ed. Tullis J. L., Academic Press, New York, pp. 143–55.

TUTTLE, W. W. and SCHOTTELIUS, B. A. (1965) *Text Book of Physiology*, 15th edn., Mosby, St. Louis.

VALENTIK, L. and WHITMORE, R. L. (1965) The terminal velocity of spheres in Bingham plastics, *Br. J. appl. Phys.* **16**, 1197–203.

VAN DEENAN, L. L. M. and DE GIER, J. (1964) Chemical composition and metabolism of lipids in red cells of various animal species, *The Red Blood Cell*, ed. Bishop, C. and Surgenor, D. M., Academic Press, New York, pp. 243–307.

VAN WAZER, J. R., LYONS, J. W., KIM, K. Y. and COLWELL, R. E. (1963) *Viscosity and Flow Measurement*, Interscience, New York.

VAND, V. (1948) Viscosity of solutions and suspensions, *J. phys. Coll. Chem.* **52**, 277–99, 300–21.

WAGNER, W. W. and FILLEY, G. F. (1963) Cinemicrography of the *in vivo* lung, *Israel J. exp. Med.* **11**, 112.

WARD, S. G. and WHITMORE, R. L. (1950) Studies of the viscosity and sedimentation of suspensions, *Br. J. appl. Phys.* **1**, 325–8.

WARNER, H. R. (1962) Use of analogue computers in the study of control mechanisms in the circulation, *Fedn. Proc., Fedn. Am. Socs. exp. Biol.* **21**, 87–91.

WAYLAND, H. and JOHNSON, P. C. (1967) Erythrocyte velocity measurement in microvessels by a correlation method, *Bibl. anat.* **2**, 160–3.

WEISS, G. H. (1964) On the theory of blood flow in tapered arteries, *Biorheol.* **2**, 153–8.

WELLS, R. E. (1964) Rheology of blood in the microvasculature, *New Engl. J. Med.* **270**, 832–9, 889–93.

WELLS, R. E. (1965) The effects of plasma proteins upon the rheology of blood in the microcirculation, *Proc. Fourth Int. Cong. on Rheol.* **4**, *Symp. on Biorheol.*, ed. Copley, A. L., Interscience, New York, pp. 431–8.

WELLS, R. E. (1967) Hemorheologic effects of the dextrans on erythrocyte aggregation, (Abstract), *Biorheol.* **4**, 88–9.

WELLS, R. E., GAWRONSKI, T. H., COX, P. J. and PERERA, R. D. (1964) Influence of fibrinogen on flow properties of erythrocyte suspensions, *Am. J. Physiol.* **207**, 1035–9.

WHITE, C. M. (1929) Streamline flow through curved pipes, *Proc. Roy. Soc.* A, **123**, 645–63.

WHITMORE, R. L. (1960a) The viscous flow of disperse suspensions in tubes, *Rheology of Disperse Systems*, ed. Mill, C. C., Pergamon, London, pp. 49–59.

WHITMORE, R. L. (1960b) Theoretical treatment of the differential flow velocities of plasma and corpuscles in living bodies, *Flow Properties of Blood*, ed. Copley, A. L. and Stainsby, G., Pergamon, London, pp. 63–81.

WHITMORE, R. L. (1963) Hemorheology and hemodynamics, *Biorheol.* **1**, 201–20.

WHITMORE, R. L. (1965a) Some flow properties of blood, *Proc. Fourth Int. Congr. on Rheol.* **1**, ed. Lee, E. H., Interscience, New York, pp. 57–71.

WHITMORE, R. L. (1965b) An application of particle/fluid mechanics to blood flow, *Proc. Fourth Int. Congr. on Rheol.* **4**, *Symp. on Biorheol.*, ed. Copley, A. L., Interscience, New York, pp. 69–82.

WHITMORE, R. L. (1966) A possible mechanism of thrombus formation, *Nature* (*London*) **209**, 298.

WHITMORE, R. L. (1967a) The Interaction forces in blood, *Bibl. anat.* **9**, 240–5.

WHITMORE, R. L. (1967b) A theory of blood flow in small vessels. *J. appl. Physiol.* **22**, 767–71.

WHITTAKER, S. R. F. and WINTON, F. R. (1933) The apparent viscosity of blood flowing in the isolated hind limb of the dog, and its variation with corpuscular concentration, *J. Physiol.* **78**, 339–69.

WIEDERHIELM, C. A. (1964) Viscoelastic properties of relaxed and constricted arteriolar walls, *Bibl. anat.* **7**, 346–52.

WIEDERHIELM, C. A. (1965) Distensibility characteristics of small blood vessels, *Fedn. Proc., Fedn. Am. Socs. exp. Biol.* **24**, 1075–84.

WIEDERHIELM, C. A. and BILLIG, L. (1967) Effects of erythrocyte orientation and concentration on light transmission through blood flowing through microscopic blood vessels, (Abstract), *Biorheol.* **4**, 99–100

WILKINSON, W. L. (1960) *Non-Newtonian Fluids*, Pergamon, London.

WINTON, F. R. and BAYLISS, L. E. (1962) *Human Physiology*, Churchill, London.

WOMBERSLEY, J. R. (1957) *An Elastic Tube Theory of Pulse Transmission and Oscillatory Flow in Mammalian Arteries*, Wright Air Dev. Center Tech. Rept. WADC-TR56-614.

YANAMI, Y., INTAGLIETTA, M., FRASHER, W. G. and WAYLAND, H. (1964) Photometric study of erythrocytes in shear flow, *Biorheol.* **2**, 165–8.

ZEDERFELDT, B. (1965) Rheological disturbances and their treatment in clinical surgery, *Proc. Fourth Int. Congr. on Rheol. 4, Symp. on Biorheol.* ed. Copley, A. L., Interscience, New York, pp. 397–408.

ZWEIFACH, B. W. and METZ, D. B. (1956) Selective distribution of blood through the terminal vascular bed of mesenteric structures and skeletal muscle, *Proc. Second Conf. on Microcirc. Physiol. and Path., Baltimore, 1955,* Williams and Wilkins, Baltimore, pp. 282–9.

INDEX